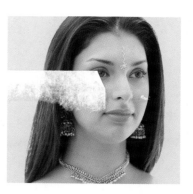

ayurveda

for beauty and health

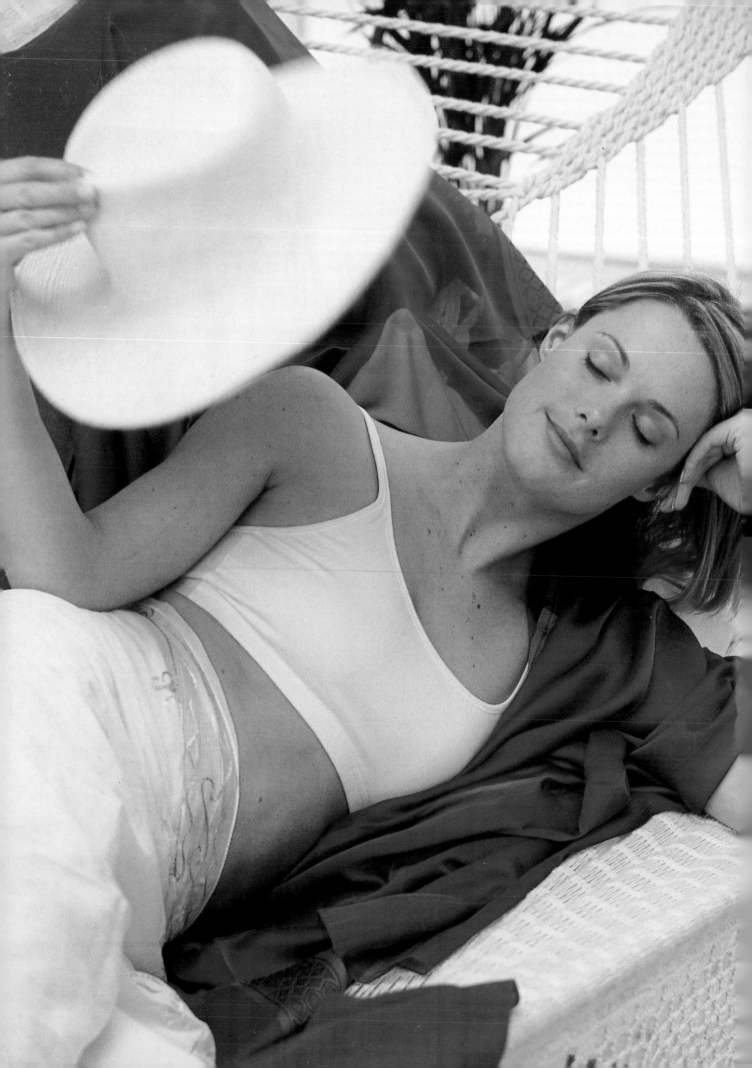

glowing fitness
and natural
well-being from
the ancient
beauty secrets
of India

ayurveda
for beauty and health

janet wright
skin-care consultant: yasmin sadikot
photographs by michelle garrett

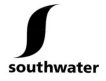

southwater

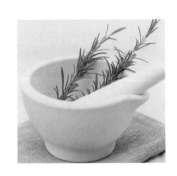

This edition is published by Southwater

Southwater is an imprint of Anness Publishing Ltd
Hermes House, 88–89 Blackfriars Road, London SE1 8HA
tel. 020 7401 2077; fax 020 7633 9499
www.southwaterbooks.com; info@anness.com

© Anness Publishing Ltd 2002, 2005

UK agent: The Manning Partnership Ltd, 6 The Old Dairy, Melcombe Road, Bath BA2 3LR;
tel. 01225 478444; fax 01225 478440; sales@manning-partnership.co.uk

UK distributor: Grantham Book Services Ltd, Isaac Newton Way, Alma Park Industrial Estate, Grantham, Lincs
NG31 9SD; tel. 01476 541080; fax 01476 541061; orders@gbs.tbs-ltd.co.uk

North American agent/distributor: National Book Network, 4501 Forbes Boulevard, Suite 200, Lanham, MD 20706;
tel. 301 459 3366; fax 301 429 5746; www.nbnbooks.com

Australian agent/distributor: Pan Macmillan Australia, Level 18, St Martins Tower, 31 Market St, Sydney, NSW 2000;
tel. 1300 135 113; fax 1300 135 103; customer.service@macmillan.com.au

New Zealand agent/distributor: David Bateman Ltd, 30 Tarndale Grove, Off Bush Road, Albany, Auckland;
tel. (09) 415 7664; fax (09) 415 8892

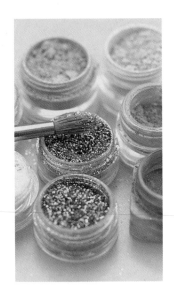

A CIP catalogue record for this book is available from the British Library.

Publisher: **Joanna Lorenz**
Project Editors: **Melanie Halton, Ann Kay**
Photographer: **Michelle Garrett**
Editorial Reader: **Penelope Goodare**

Editorial Director: **Helen Sudell**
Designer: **Ann Cannings**
Copy Editor: **Beverley Jollands**
Production Controller: **Claire Rae**

Previously published as *Ayurvedic Beauty*

10 9 8 7 6 5 4 3 2 1

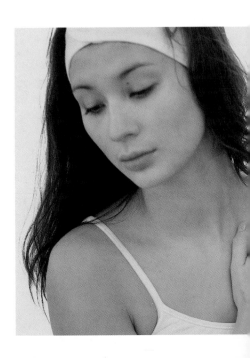

Note to reader:
The reader should not regard the recommendations, ideas and techniques expressed and described
in this book as substitutes for the advice of a qualified medical practitioner or other qualified
professional. Any use to which the recommendations, ideas and techniques are put is at the
reader's sole discretion and risk.

Contents

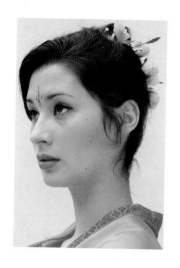

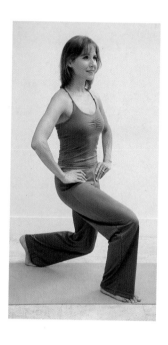

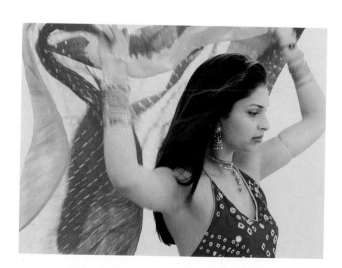

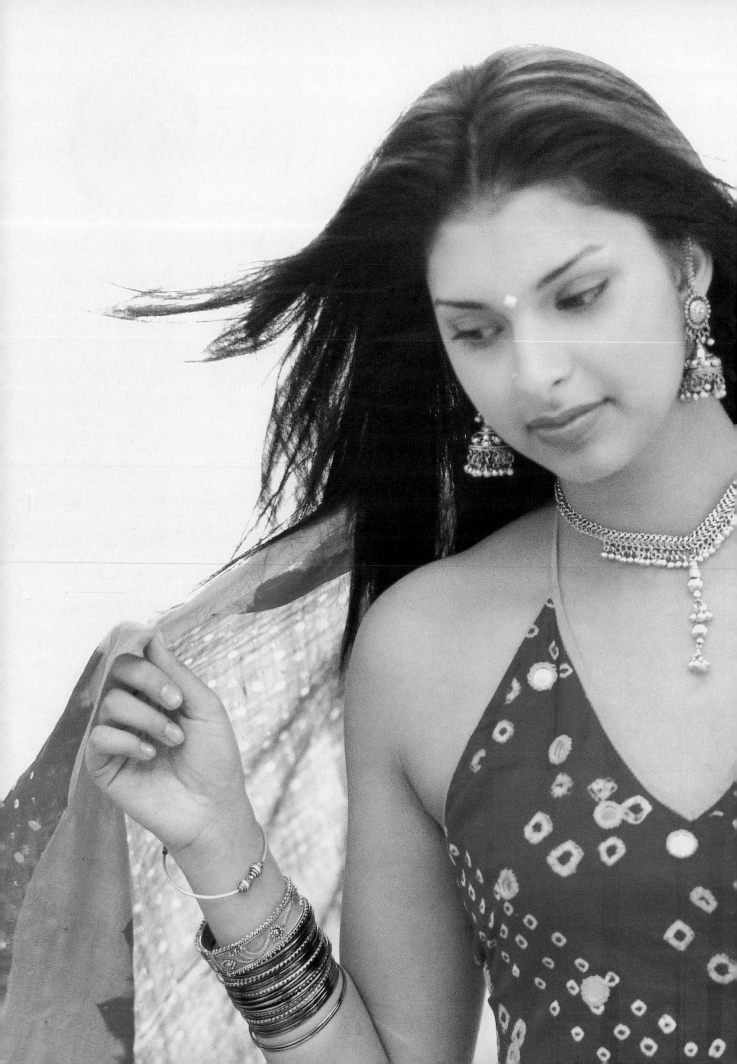

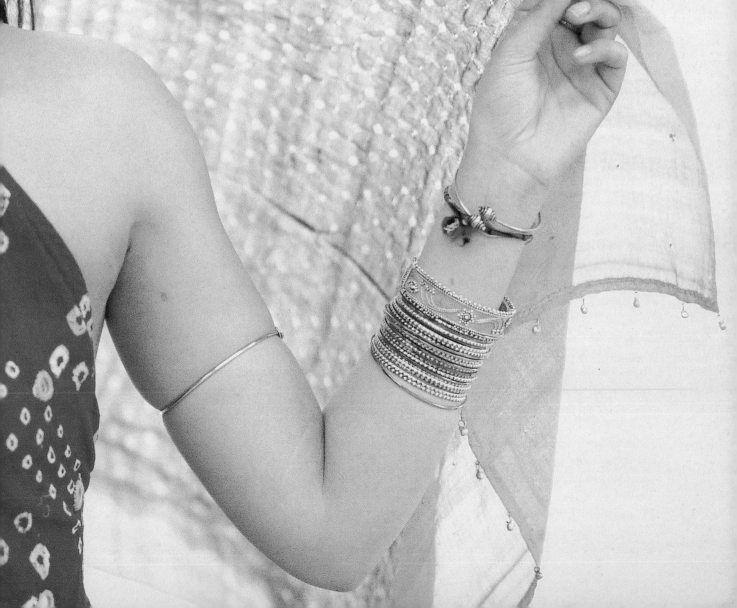

The Spirit of Ayurveda

Ayurveda offers grace, vitality and serenity: it is a tradition that values beauty as a sign of inner harmony. India's Ayurvedic health system is several thousand years old, yet in the 21st century it is being taken up enthusiastically by people all over the world.

A tradition of beauty

Ayurveda, the "science of life", is a philosophy that covers every aspect of being: health, food, spirit, sex, occupation and relationships. It teaches how to live in harmony with your inner self and with the world around you. At one extreme of this far-reaching philosophy are the practices of religious ascetics, who subject themselves to fasts and other rigours to try to transcend the physical. At the other extreme are the sensual paintings, sculptures and writings that reveal a people at ease with their bodies and appreciative of the pleasures of life.

beauty of body and soul

For both men and women, beauty is seen as a blessing in India: gods and goddesses, heroes and heroines are depicted as handsome and graceful, with arched eyebrows and delicate features, and images of women's beauty and vigour appear in the earliest sacred texts. Traditionally, Indian women have adorned themselves with jewellery, make-up and body art. They have perfumed their hair and dressed it with flowers and gems. They have worn garments in dazzling colours, choosing fitted blouses that emphasize body shape, or swirling saris that draw attention to graceful movement.

Both sexes have traditionally groomed themselves to make the most of their looks. Since the earliest times, Ayurvedic remedies have included techniques to brighten eyes, clear skin and enhance the lustre of hair. Anti-aging treatments are among the most popular, aimed at restoring not only physical vigour but also a youthful appearance.

Because the philosophy of Ayurveda treats body, mind and soul as interrelated, beauty is not limited to the physical dimension, but reflects the vitality and health of the whole person, and adornment plays only a minor part. Jewels are valued not only for their beauty but also because they are considered to possess health-enhancing properties. Herbal remedies and treatments aim to cleanse the body from the

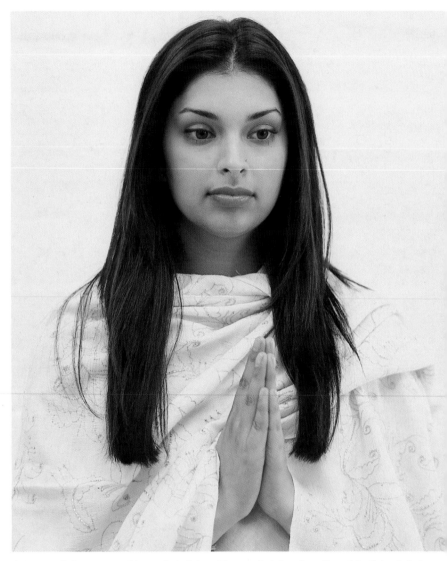

△ **Harmony is the essence of Ayurveda. India's goddesses of wisdom, love, life and death teach their followers to blend action with reflection, courage with compassion, so beauty grows from inner radiance.**

inside, while meditative practices prevent stress leaving its mark, and a fitness regime ensures agelessly youthful physical grace.

Ayurvedic medicine

Some of the basic principles of Ayurveda were set out more than 3,000 years ago in the Vedas, the sacred texts of Hinduism, and its teachings are believed to have been passed on by word of mouth for many centuries before that. The earliest medical textbooks, the *Susruta Samhita* and the *Charaka Samhita* (written before 500 BC and still consulted

today), list more than 700 herbal medicine 125 surgical instruments and a range of procedures including cosmetic surgery and kidney-stone removal. Human bone excavated from the city of Harappa, dating from before 1500 BC, bear evidence of surgical repairs.

In the ancient world, Ayurveda influence spread as far as Egypt, China and Greece. Since Western medicine developed from that of the ancient Greeks, a trace of Ayurveda survives in modern medical training, for example in kidney operation nd the diagnosis of eye disease. In most ways, modern medicine has diverged from lder traditions, focusing on symptoms and pecific diseases, but now, when the healing ower of antibiotics is waning because of veruse, and other wonder drugs have evealed harmful side-effects, the ancient visdom of traditional holistic healing ystems is again being sought. Western nedicine is starting to open its mind, dmitting that some treatments work in vays that no one understands and that mind nd body can work together to heal illness.

Meanwhile, Ayurvedic researchers are ublishing impressive results in mainstream nedical journals. In one study, a remedy alled gugalipid, made of resin from the nyrrh tree, was found to lower cholesterol levels by an average of 20 per cent. In another, doctors reported that the skin condition of patients using an Ayurvedic remedy improved noticeably, while a placebo had no such results.

balance and harmony

The principle of Ayurveda is that good health stems from a correct balance of different energies and harmony with the outside world. As a medical system it is holistic, and though remedies exist for specific problems, they are varied according to the person.

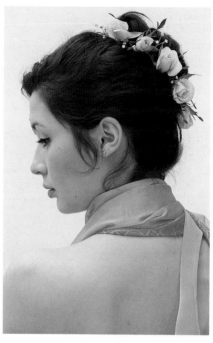

△ Jewellery and ornament symbolize some of the links between the worlds of body and spirit.

▽ **A traditional exercise regime and an active lifestyle can allow every woman to achieve the natural grace of a classical dancer.**

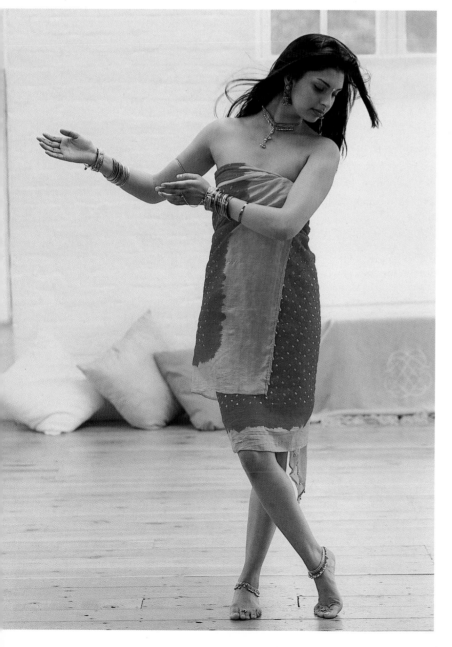

Ayurveda also works on levels other than the physical, and this is where it differs most radically from Western medicine. It is part of a world-view that accepts the existence of the unseen, both as part of a human being (a non-physical body that overlaps with the physical one) and as external energies that can affect us. Ayurveda makes no division between science and religion, so its medical system places at least as much emphasis on the psychological and spiritual as on the physical. Most treatments are intended to bring disturbed energies back into balance, allowing the body to heal itself.

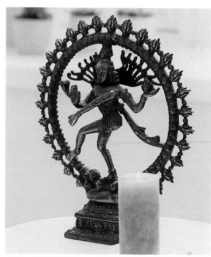

△ Prayer and meditation may help as much as herbal remedies when health disorders indicate that vital energies have been disturbed.

Living energies, healing powers

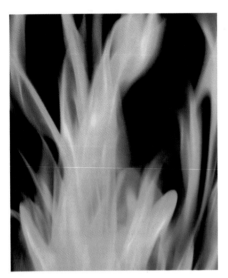

△ Fire is one of the five elemental forces present in the whole of creation, including ourselves.

According to Ayurveda, five *mahabhutas* or "great elements" – air, fire, water, earth, and ether (or space) – constitute the world with everything in it, including ourselves, and they affect us through three primary forces called *doshas* (meaning "flaws"): *vata*, *pitta* and *kapha*. Each dosha owes its character to the elements associated with it:

• Vata, linked with the elements air and ether, is dry. It governs movement of every kind, both mental and physical.

• Pitta, linked with fire and water, is hot. It governs all the processes of change and transformation, such as digestion.

• Kapha, linked with earth and water, is heavy. It governs structure and stability.

channels of energy

The doshas are not the only forces that affect us, because our non-physical body has its own detailed anatomy. Just as the blood carries oxygen around the body, another equally essential life force called *prana* circulates in channels of its own. At any junction – for example where two kinds of tissue meet, such as bone and tendon, or where the influences of two energies meet – there are *marma points*, where energy sometimes gets blocked. One of the major energy channels follows the line of the backbone and is studded with seven important points called *chakras*.

The physical and non-physical constantly overlap. For example, *ama*, a toxin formed in the body, can be created by poorly digested food or by an experience you can't assimilate – or swallow. *Ojas*, the subtle energy that connects body, mind and spirit, both creates our aura and underpins the immune system. It is formed from the seven kinds of body tissue, and is also influenced by meditation.

imbalance

We are born in a state called *prakruti*, with all three doshas in balance though not in equal amounts. Each of us is governed by one more than the others, and our individual natures mean that even with the energies comfortably in balance, we'll show the attributes of the dominant dosha. Problems begin when one dosha becomes excessively powerful, pushing us to extremes of behaviour or creating ill-health. Excessive vata might cause anxiety or a hacking cough. Too much fiery pitta could trigger an attack of road rage or heartburn.

Stolid kapha could bring everything to standstill, resulting in anything from lethargy to blocked sinuses. To prevent remedy such problems, Ayurveda aims maintain balance in all things. That includ keeping people in harmony with the surroundings and with each other, keepin bodily processes working effectively, an keeping body, mind and spirit integrated.

Sometimes imbalance results from a excess of one of the doshas, perhaps becau we're eating the wrong kinds of food. C we could be affected by something we'v come into contact with, since everythin has one of three *gunas*, or inner qualitie harmonious *sattva*, aggressive *rajas* or du *tamas*. Anything from foods to colours thoughts will do us good if it's sattvic, but likely to cause irritation if it's rajasic heaviness if it's tamasic. The problem cou even be caused by karma: the result misdeeds in this life or a previous one.

Ayurvedic therapies

All Ayurvedic treatment is aimed restoring balance, in order to keep us stron enough – both in spirit and in immun system – to withstand disease, so it is used f

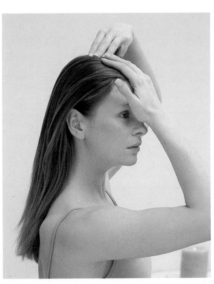

△ To locate the crown marma point, rest one hand on the bridge of your nose and measure three fingerwidths back from your fingertips.

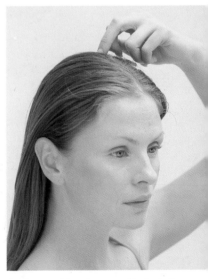

△ Massage this point to get blocked energy moving on if you are suffering from a feeling of confusion.

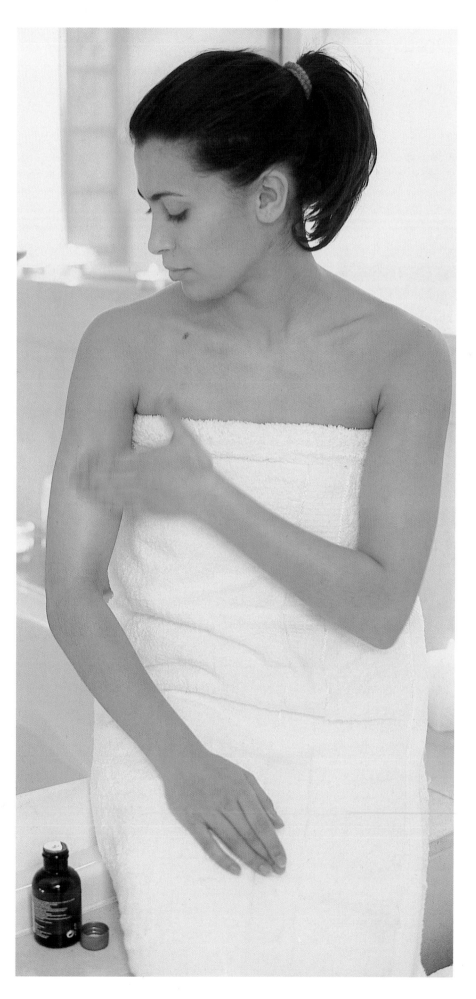

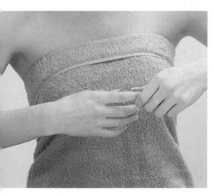

> Ayurveda recommends regular detoxifying treatments, starting with steam baths and herbal oil massage. Spring is a good time to initiate these cleansing practices.

prevention as well as for cure. Massage, yoga and meditation form part of Ayurveda's recommended daily routine, but can also be used to treat certain health problems.

Nutrition is one of Ayurveda's central elements, with the emphasis not only on wholesome ingredients but also on the right foods for you as an individual. Each dosha can be aggravated by certain foods, so if you're suffering from an imbalance, you'll be urged to avoid those foods and eat others that have a calming effect.

Detoxification, or *shodhana*, begins with *purvakarma*: cleansing steam baths and herbal oil massages. Then comes *panchakarma*, a more rigorous detox that may include enemas, laxatives, and nasal washes with herbs or oils. In case blocked energy is causing congestion, the marma points may be stimulated to encourage the flow. This is usually done with finger pressure, though needles may also be used.

The next step, *rasayana*, aims to restore long-term health and slow down the aging process through lifestyle changes, meditation and exercises, with herbal remedies if necessary. A course of treatment may last for up to six months.

Though some of Ayurveda's practices seem strenuous, it's a compassionate philosophy that understands human desires and aims to increase the quality of life, promoting vitality and inner harmony.

△ Hand massage stimulates the marma points that are clustered in this area, and it is easy to do it for yourself.

Dosha analysis

If you consult an Ayurvedic doctor you may be asked to complete a questionnaire to find out your *prakruti* – your constitution, determined at the time of your birth – and your current imbalance, or *vikruti*. The questionnaire is part of a package of diagnostic tools; others include checking your pulses (subtle energy flows) and examining the condition of your tongue. Answering a questionnaire at home can give you an idea of your vikruti, as your answers will usually be based on your current condition, but it does not replace a full consultation with a practitioner.

You may find that more than one description applies to you. In this case, tick all that are relevant. In the skin and hair sections, respond only to the descriptions that apply to you. Give yourself plenty of time to think before answering, so your answers will be as accurate as possible.

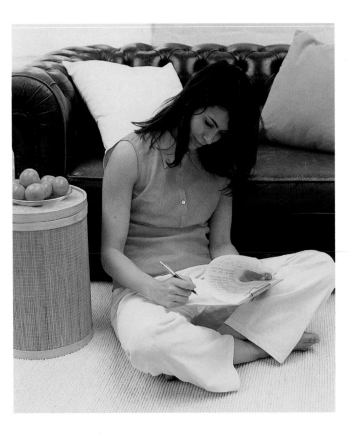

◁ **Completing a questionnaire can give some insight into your current needs, so make sure your answers reflect the way you're feeling right now.**

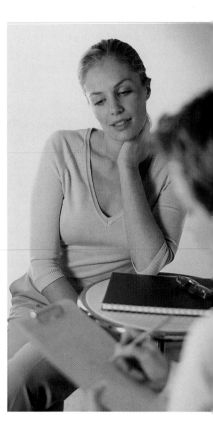

▷ **To discover your true constitution – the state in which you were born – you'll need to consult an Ayurvedic practitioner. The results may surprise you.**

dosha analysis

PHYSICAL TRAITS	VATA	PITTA	KAPHA
Body frame	Thin	Medium	Large
Fingernails	Thin/cracking	Pink/soft/medium	Thick/wide/pale
Weight	Low/bony	Medium/muscular	Gains easily
Stool/bowel movement	Small/hard/wind	Loose/burning	Moderate/solid
Forehead size	Small	Medium	Large
Appetite	Variable	Strong	Constant
Eyes	Small/unsteady	Reddish/focused	Wide/white
Voice	Low or weak	High or sharp	Slow or quiet
Lips	Cracking, thin, dry	Medium or soft	Large or smooth
Speech	Quick or talkative	Moderate or argumentative	Deep or melodious
Weather: what bothers you?	Cold and dry	Heat and sun	Cold and damp
Sleep patterns	Light	Moderate	Deep/heavy
Which do you like best?	Travel or nature	Sports or politics	Water or flowers

MENTAL TRAITS	VATA	PITTA	KAPHA
Temperament	Nervous or fearful	Irritable or impatient	Easy-going
Memory	Quickly grasps, but forgets	Sharp or clear	Slow to learn, never forgets
Faith	Radical or changing	Leader- or goal-oriented	Loyal or constant
Dreams	Flying or anxious	Fighting or in colour	Few or romantic
Emotions	Enthusiastic or worried	Warm or angry	Calm or attached
Mind	Quick or adaptable	Penetrating or critical	Slow and steady

SKIN TENDENCIES	VATA	PITTA	KAPHA
	Lack of tone or lustre	Rashes, inflammation, itching	Dull, sluggish, congested
	Rough patches	Oily T-zone	Enlarged pores
	Chapping and cracking	Premature wrinkling	Large pustules
	Dry eczema	Blackheads	Cystic formations
	General dryness	General excessive oiliness	Thick, oily secretions
	Dandruff/dry scalp	Discoloration	Oily scalp
			Strong, flawless
	Fine, porcelain	Warm, smooth	

HAIR	VATA	PITTA	KAPHA
	Dry and dull	Oily	Thick
	Frizzy	Balding	Glossy
	Scaly scalp	Excessive hair loss	Shiny
	Split ends	Thinning	Grows easily

▽ Vata is a fine, light, speedy energy that can cause problems with dryness of skin and hair.

▽ If pitta's fiery warmth slips out of balance, it may express itself in rashes and discoloration.

▽ Kapha's strong skin and thick hair age slowly; excess oiliness is the main beauty pitfall.

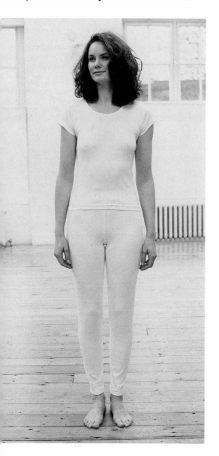

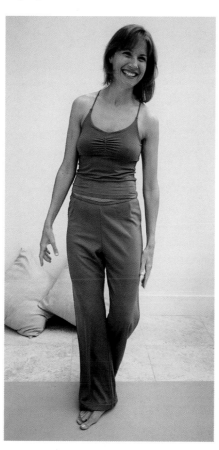

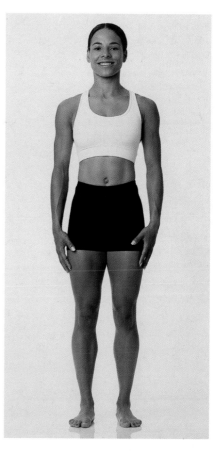

Your dosha and you

Few people are ruled by a single dosha. Most of us are governed by dual doshas, one of which is more powerful than the other. A very few are ruled equally by all three.

If your score in the questionnaire is highest in pitta but still quite high in kapha, for example, that makes you a pitta-kapha combination. Scores reversed for pitta and kapha would make you a kapha-pitta. The pitta-kapha person is more likely to suffer from a pitta imbalance than anything else. But a combination of factors that aggravate kapha – such as eating a lot of heavy food during a cold, damp spring – could produce an excess of kapha energy.

self-analysis

The results of the questionnaire can be enlightening. If they are puzzling because they seem unlike you, your answers to the questions may not have been completely accurate: perhaps you overstated your faults or gave answers you felt ought to be true. You may be used to thinking of yourself in a way that is no longer relevant.

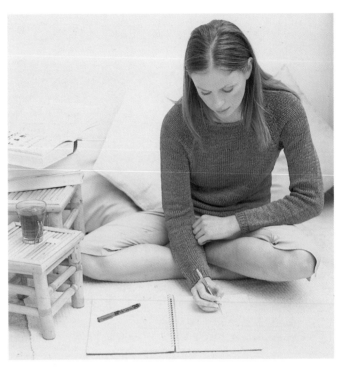

◁ Vata dominates the afternoon hours, making this a good time for thought and intellectual activity, rather than physical work.

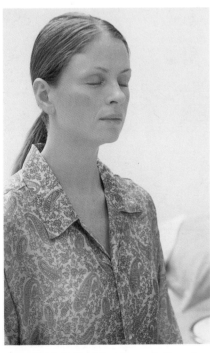

△ Morning is the best time for meditation, when peaceful kapha energy helps to still your mind.

Comparisons should be made with other people of your own ethnic background, not against some kind of world average. Kapha, for example, tends to go with fair skin and vata with dark skin. But a typical kapha person from Sri Lanka would be darker than, say, a typical vata from Sweden.

Remember too that your mind and body may be ruled by different doshas, so you might have a fiery pitta temperament in a curvy kapha body. All kinds of external factors can affect you: even the season or weather could influence your answers. So don't feel ruled by the results you obtain. They are meant to offer guidance, not lay down the law.

In order to discover your prakruti, or constitutional dosha, an Ayurvedic practitioner will carry out a pulse analysis, taking the pulses of the subtle energy flows at 21 points. The difference between your prakruti and your vikruti can be revealing. Prakruti is your ideal state, with everything in the best balance for your personality – if there's a big difference it could mean you're living in a way that doesn't suit you.

what is an imbalance?

We all have one or two doshas that dominate. It's natural for each of us to show some characteristics of these, whether they are most noticeable in our looks, behaviour or tastes. The doshas also give us warning of what needs to be tackled if something goes wrong with our well-being.

When a dominant dosha becomes excessively strong, its characteristics are exaggerated. As a pitta type you will be naturally ambitious and competitive, for example, but if pitta grows too strong you may become irritable and critical, and have trouble sleeping. This is known as a pitta imbalance. If you don't tackle an imbalance

THE DOSHAS THROUGH THE DAY	
6am–10am	Kapha
10am–2pm	Pitta
2pm–6pm	Vata
6pm–10pm	Kapha
10pm–2am	Pitta
2am–6am	Vata

early on, it can eventually manifest itself in sickness, so you need to reduce your dominant dosha. In this case, that means cutting down on things like spicy food and dance music, which fuel pitta.

a time for everything

According to Ayurvedic teaching, each period of the day is ruled by a different energy, which can reinforce or counteract the influence of your dominant dosha.

Tranquil kapha governs early morning, the time for meditation. Later in the morning is the time to exercise, combining kapha strength with pitta energy. Pitta, which aids digestion, rules midday, making that the best time to eat. Vata dominates the afternoon – an ideal time for mental work, as vata promotes intelligence. Then come the quiet kapha hours again, making this the best time to get to sleep. Pitta takes over again after 10pm, when its fiery energy is meant to stop your temperature dropping too low while you sleep. If you go to bed after 10pm, you may find that a new rush of pitta-fuelled energy stops you dropping off.

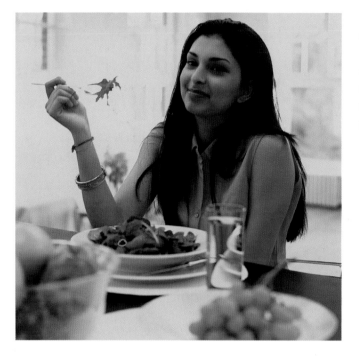

◁ Pitta energy, which aids digestion, is in full force around lunchtime, making this the best time to enjoy your main meal of the day.

▽ Ayurveda advocates "early to bed, early to rise". Before 10pm, kapha helps you to get to sleep – after that, pitta could keep you awake.

The seasons follow the same rhythm as the hours of the day, with kapha ruling the weeks from spring to early summer, pitta ruling high summer and autumn, and vata rising when the leaves have fallen to dominate the winter.

Since an excess of any dosha brings out its harmful side, watch out for signs of an imbalance, especially during the times or seasons that correspond with your own dominant dosha. You might find it hard to drag yourself out of bed in the kapha-ruled morning, or that pitta's summer heat brings you out in a rash, or that you're getting stressed under vata's influence during the winter months. Medical researchers have found that seasonal affective disorder, or "winter blues", actually affects most people during spring, when depressive kapha is coming into force.

Even our own lives follow these phases. As children we are ruled by kapha, as adults pitta takes over and with the onset of wise old age we come into our vata time.

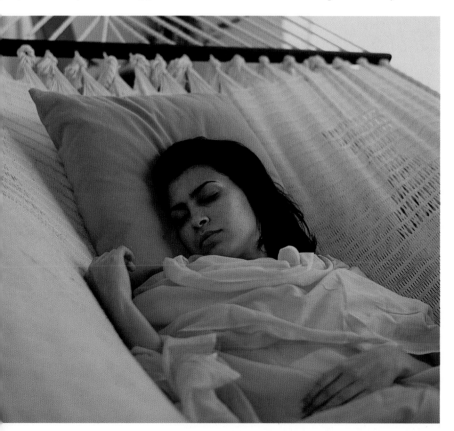

ESSENTIAL FLAWS

Why are the forces of vata, pitta and kapha called doshas, or "flaws"? Ayurveda takes the very practical view that, though everything ought to exist in perfect balance, it usually doesn't. Our individual natures dictate that one dosha will generally be dominant, and this is fine when it is just enough to express your individual personality, but when it becomes too strong and overrules the others, it throws your constitution out of balance, which leads to ill health. So a healthy life is one in which we manage to keep the balance steady.

Vata movement and life force

Slender, willowy and long-legged, the classic vata woman looks good on a catwalk. She's more likely to be either tall or petite than of medium height. Her cool, porcelain skin is rarely bothered by spots or oily patches. Her rather small eyes sparkle with life and intelligence, and her fine hair complements her delicate bone structure.

She never thinks about her weight – she's naturally light. Her active lifestyle keeps her in shape, and she doesn't tend to eat a lot. She'd rather be in a club, dancing until dawn, than wasting time in a restaurant where you can't move to the music. Though a born athlete, she rarely builds a lot of muscle, but remains slim and slightly ethereal-looking.

as free as the air

Vata women love change, travel and movement. They're fast – whether they're running for the sheer joy of it or tackling some new concept in a physics class. They talk rapidly and their quick intellects mean they're full of ideas, plans and theories.

At work, vatas are the ones with all the ideas who'll get any project under way with the force of their enthusiasm, though they may not be so good at seeing it through: while someone with a steadier dosha takes over, they'll be hatching a dozen new plans. They're highly creative and often artistic, so no one really expects them to be utterly practical. They'd be exhausting company if they weren't so stimulating, but they rarely stay long enough to wear out their welcome.

vata imbalance

No one can keep up that pace for ever. Vatas are smart enough to know this, but often don't slow down until they've built up a massive vata imbalance by doing all the things that aggravate this ethereal dosha. These include skipping meals, not getting enough sleep and generally running themselves into the ground.

When vatas finally crash they may have trouble getting up again. Then they suffer

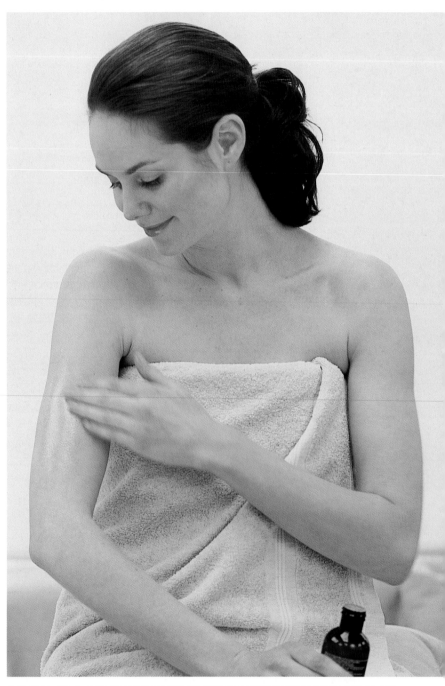

△ **Soothing oils do more than just nourish dry skin: they can help pacify excess vata energy.**

from stress and exhaustion, probably compounded by insomnia. Living on their nerves, they can forget to eat or may feel too anxious to swallow anything. Their rapid intellect can spin off into confusion. Tension can lead to muscle pain, cramps and irritable bowel syndrome. Excessive weight loss can also lead to serious health problem such as osteoporosis.

Dryness is the essential vata attribute, so an excess of vata causes dehydration in everything: hair and fingernails become brittle, lips crack, the tongue feels like felt the eyes are sore. Dry skin conditions such a

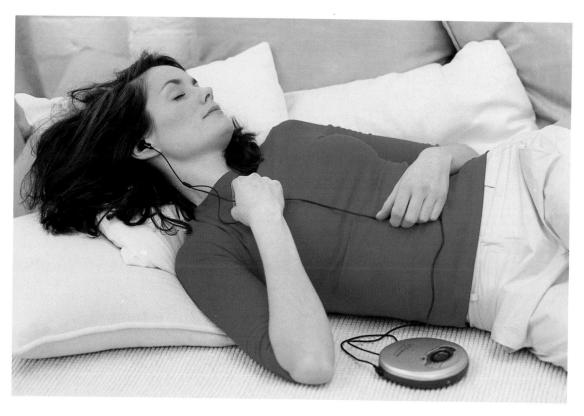

◁ Listening to classical music with a slow, rhythmic beat can help to calm a vata imbalance, easing away feelings of tension and anxiety.

eczema can be a problem. A dry cough adds to the feeling of debility. Internal dryness can cause arthritis and constipation and even thicken the blood – add this to vata's raised stress levels, and it's not surprising that high blood pressure and heart palpitations are vata complaints.

pacifying vata

This dosha needs help to become more grounded. Pacifying influences are warm, moist, slow and contained. If you're vata, you're drawn towards speed, lightness, novelty. Try to balance these with activities that slow and centre you. Take a relaxing spa break instead of a strenuous activity holiday and discover the steam room and the jacuzzi. Listen to peaceful New Age or classical music. Find a course in meditation, then practise it at home some mornings instead of heading for the gym for your normal workout.

You like being with people, but this doesn't have to be in a crowded club. Invite friends around for supper instead. Take your time selecting wonderful ingredients, cooking the meal to perfection and eating it with people who care about you. Relax and enjoy the warmth of their company.

Cold, dry, windy weather makes you tense, so cocoon yourself away from it when

you can, and take your holidays on a tropical beach. Even the scents you use can fuel or calm your dosha: jasmine, sandalwood and rose all help to keep vata in balance.

your beauty needs

Dry skin is the classic vata complaint. The fine texture of your skin looks good when vata is in balance, but an imbalance makes it dull and lifeless. This kind of skin ages easily, so moisturizing is vital: the Ayurvedic way is to drink lots of water and eat plenty of the juicy fruits that help to pacify vata. Putting on weight isn't a problem for this dosha, so

you should never really need to count any calories, but you do need to beware of letting your weight fall too low.

Vata's flyaway hair is prone to dandruff, so a weekly sesame oil massage will relieve your dry scalp as well as easing tension. Teeth are a weak spot, exacerbated by the vata tendency to graze instead of eating meals, leaving teeth constantly coated in acid. If you can't cut out the snacks, rinse your mouth with water after every one.

▽ As a vata, you love company, and a leisurely meal with a friend will help you relax.

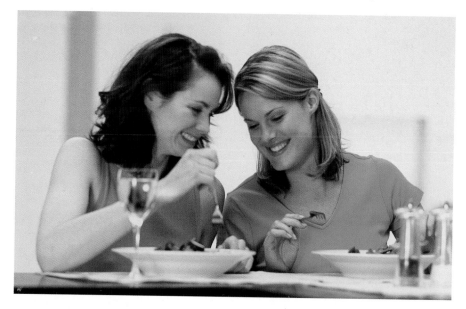

Pitta fire and transformation

Pitta woman is a dazzler. Fire is her dominant element, and it shows. Women of this dosha radiate energy like the sun, and their skin reflects their emotions with a surge of colour. Yet pitta also includes an element of water, which can stop this dosha burning out.

Despite a healthy appetite, pittas rarely become overweight. You're likely to spot them at the gym, where their powerful workouts result in toned muscles that curve rather than bulking up. They are usually blessed with soft hair, neat noses and small chins, and may have numerous beauty spots in the form of moles and freckles.

Though they're likely to have combination skin – with an oilier T-zone of forehead, nose and mouth – as long as pitta remains in balance the skin should be neither too dry nor too oily, but smooth and warm to the touch. Pittas often have warm, coppery skin tones.

fiery energies

The heat extends to the pitta character. Passionate and ambitious, pitta women know what they want and will strive to achieve it. They may fly off the handle, but they're not the sort to hide a simmering grievance behind a mask of friendliness. Don't be fooled by this fiery image, though. As long as pitta remains in balance, they are intelligent, calm and rational. Born leaders, their qualities reward those who are drawn to their fire.

At work, they're high-fliers, strong-minded and focused: if they're enthusiastic about a project they'll see it through. They aim for the heights of success and often reach them, thanks to the single-minded work they put into getting there.

pitta imbalance

When pitta energy boils over, the heat is on. Rashes, inflammation, sweating, fevers and heartburn are all signs of a pitta imbalance, as are acne eruptions and hot flushes, which characterize the beginning and end of the fertile life period ruled by this fiery dosha.

A pitta imbalance will often reveal itself through the skin, in blotching or changes in pigmentation, or the flushing caused by indigestion. More serious ailments may be signalled by a yellowish complexion: this could be caused by liver dysfunction, which needs medical attention.

Fiery mood swings may be caused by another of pitta's problems – hormone imbalances. An excess of pitta can make someone overambitious, temperamental, jealous, aggressive and likely to trample on anyone in their path.

pacifying pitta

Your inner fire provides all the heat you need. Sultry weather and overheated buildings can provoke a pitta imbalance. When you go to the gym, head for the swimming pool rather than the sauna or hot tub. On holiday, go for the snow. In the summer, slow down to keep cool. The

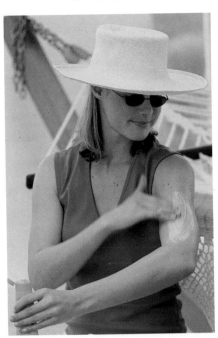

◁ **Use sunscreen at all times to protect yourself from the sun (and be sure to avoid sunbeds), especially if you have moles or freckles.**

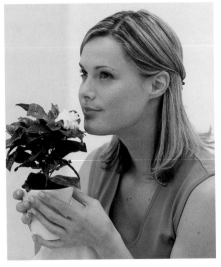

△ **If excessive pitta energy makes you irritable, soothe yourself with gentle influences: the scent of a gardenia, the sound of trickling water.**

influences that pacify excess pitta are cool, soft, kind and generally calming. The smell of gardenias is meant to cool pitta energy.

Give yourself time to eat breakfast and lunch sitting down, instead of skipping meals and overdosing on food in the evening. This can help you to avoid the pitta pitfalls of insomnia and indigestion, which add to your stress.

Avoid harsh or aggressive music, or anything with a driving beat or lots of drumming. Try soothing music with a slowish beat and gentle, minor chords.

Since high-tech equipment also increases pitta energy, an overheated office can cause problems. Freelance work can be one solution, keeping you away from office politics. On the other hand, being part of a team could help control your tendency to overwork. Whichever you choose, keep an eye on your stress levels and remember there's a world outside work. Cultivate friends who help you relax rather than contacts who can advance your career. Use some of your abundant creativity to express your artistic gifts, and divert some energy into working for a good cause that gives you a feelgood buzz.

your beauty needs

Ruled by fire, your skin reacts readily to inner or outer heat. You flush when you are angry and blush with embarrassment. Indigestion may give you an unwanted glow, and hot conditions make you look and feel uncomfortable. Colour-reducing foundation creams were made for you.

Your skin is sensitive, and a pitta imbalance can bring you out in rashes, rosacea, acne or – in later life – blotchy liver spots. Dark-skinned pittas sometimes suffer from pigmented patches. Your most important beauty rule is to keep cool. A mineral-water spray lives in your handbag or desk drawer; at home, cucumber makes an instant skin-cooling mask. Treat your skin kindly, avoiding harsh treatments that could bring it out in a rash.

Your skin isn't dry and shouldn't age too fast, as long as you protect it from the sun. It's lucky that pitta's sensitive skin and dislike of heat tend to stop you sunbathing, because you're more prone than anyone else to skin cancer. Keep an eye on all those moles, reporting any changes to your doctor.

A pitta imbalance can also affect your hair, making it prematurely thin and grey. Ayurvedic hair care aims at keeping the scalp healthy and strengthening growth.

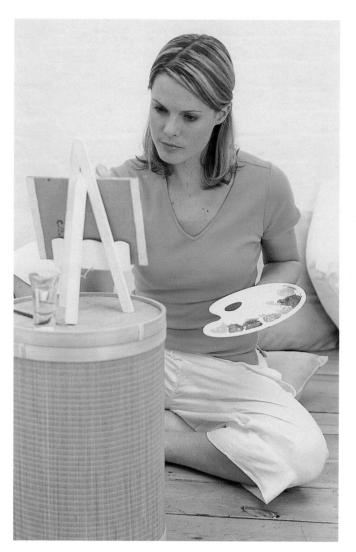

◁ To keep your life in balance, put some of your abundant pitta energy into expressing your natural creativity.

▽ Calm pitta heat with a refreshing spray of cool water – it's good for your skin, and for your equilibrium – or, even better, go for a swim.

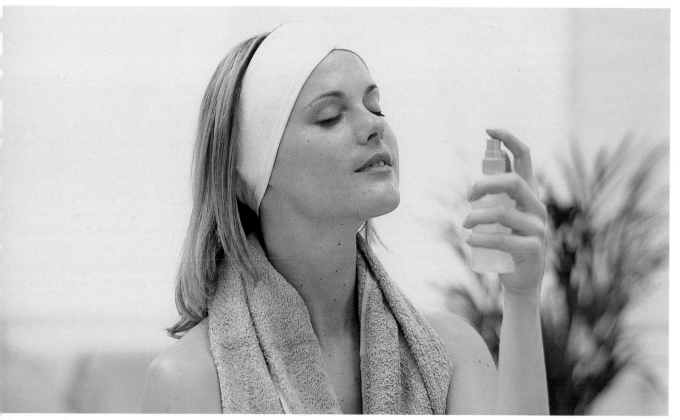

Kapha growth and protection

A classic kapha type has perfect teeth, full lips and a flawless complexion, surrounded by masses of shining hair. But her greatest beauty shines out through her eyes, which are large, deep and thickly fringed with long eyelashes. The inner quality they reveal is one of peace and serenity. Kapha's very presence is calming, and the stress that aggravates vata's dizziness and pitta's temper seems to dissipate when a kapha person takes over. This is a peaceful, stable energy, combining earth's strength with water's deep stillness. Kapha people relax easily and rarely experience a troubled night.

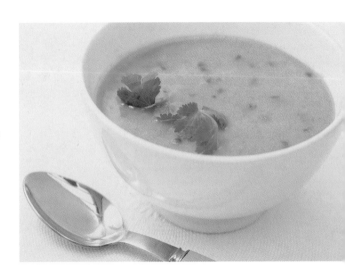

▷ **Sensual kaphas appreciate the pleasures of food, but this can lead to weight gain. Spicy soups and curries will satisfy your tastebuds and pacify excess kapha energy.**

peace from earth

Calm and tolerant, kaphas are natural peace-makers. They make friends easily, love deeply and are wise enough to forgive things that would offend others. They happily nurture those they love, and frequently all those around them too, maintaining deep, rewarding relationships of all kinds. They are outstanding homemakers, and will go to great lengths to avoid change or upheaval.

At work they defuse tense situations with their down-to-earth good humour. In fact, tension is less likely to develop when there are kapha people around to carry a burden, because they are both physically and psychologically strong, with legendary powers of endurance. On a practical level they'll finish the work that airy vatas started and lost interest in – and they won't be drawn into arguments with a bossy pitta. Good memory, aided by their natural patience, helps them stay on course and get the details right.

All sorts of people are drawn toward kapha's sweetness and warmth. Kaphas are too kind to reject anyone, but they have to beware of a tendency to let more demanding types take advantage.

kapha imbalance

In excess, grounded kapha energy can become heavy and stagnant. Kapha people relax very easily, and have to battle with their lazy tendencies. When kapha starts to overrule everything else, it's hard to get them off the sofa.

Exercise is vital to keep kapha energy at a healthy level, but lethargy may be a sign of another characteristic problem: depression. A kapha person in low spirits will tend to stay at home eating chocolate in front of the television: negative traits combining to increase the imbalance.

Groundedness can also distort into materialism, and when that happens, greed

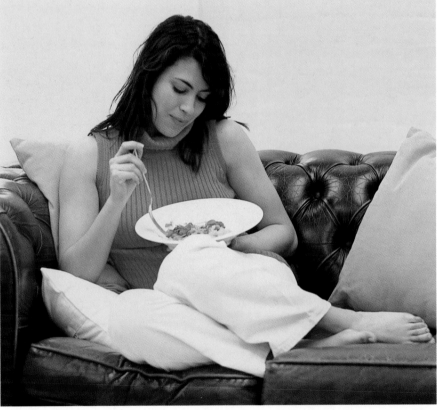

◁ **Lethargy can be a problem for kaphas, especially when they are bored or lonely.**

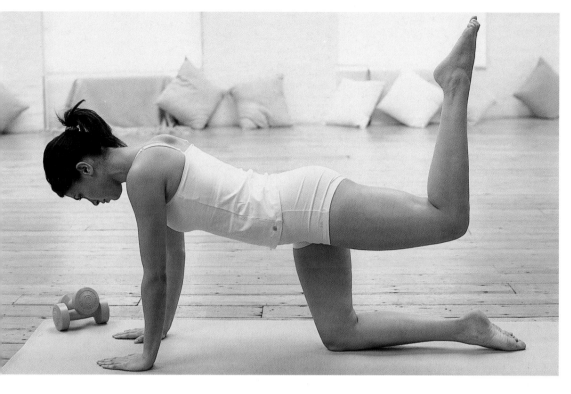

◁ Kaphas have to push themselves to exercise, but the ease with which they develop muscles is encouraging. They also need to work on flexibility and lightness.

21

the spirit of ayurveda

and envy are kapha's less appealing traits, along with a possessive attachment to material things. A kapha overdose has a blunting, dulling effect on mental faculties, leading to obstinacy and narrow-mindedness. Physically, it is associated with sluggish digestion, constipation, respiratory congestion, diabetes, coronary artery disease, slowed metabolism and obesity.

pacifying kapha

You probably love rich food, sweet or savoury, and plenty of it. But that increases kapha energy as well as your hip measurement. If you're becoming greedy or sluggish, try some hot, spicy food for a change, and eat a bit less. Brisk scents such as cedar or camphor can sometimes help, as does anything that has a tendency to lighten, warm or invigorate.

Kapha people need to get up early and take daily exercise. If you're sleeping more than eight hours a night (nine in your teens), get your doctor to check for an underactive thyroid gland. Depression can also make you oversleep; to break the cycle, find an activity you can enjoy in company: team sports, walking or aerobics classes with a friend.

You need to stay stimulated, so seek new experiences and motivate yourself to go out to evening classes or art galleries. Put aside your cookbook and read a history of your

area, a thriller (make sure you solve the mystery before it's all revealed), or a biography of someone you admire.

Coldness increases kapha, so work up a sweat in the gym and enjoy the sauna too – not the steam room, because you need dry heat. Slap on the sunscreen and go out on sunny days. Take an outdoor holiday visiting archaeological sites in the North African

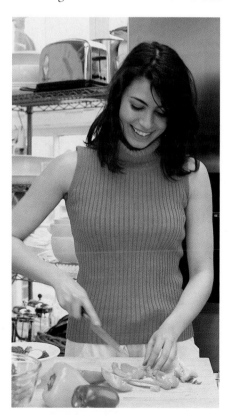

desert or exploring the Australian outback. Let your nurturing tendencies do yourself some good and adopt an unwanted dog: you're too kind-hearted to neglect the long walks it'll need.

your beauty needs

Kaphas have the sort of strong, smooth skin that shrugs off most blemishes and goes on to age well. Your idea of a bad-hair day would win no sympathy from anyone else.

What you have to watch out for is your weight. You're naturally strong and fit, so the health benefits of exercise aren't much of a draw. You enjoy life's little indulgences, such as good food, warmth and relaxation. A run down to the gym on a cold night sounds as much fun to you as drilling your own teeth.

The strongest of the doshas, you build muscle easily, so you'll see easy gains when you start working out. You'll need to cut down your fuel intake as well. But if you eat at the right time – just long enough before exercise to give you the energy you need without risking indigestion – you'll find working out doesn't make you overeat in compensation. Then your honed physique will start to offer its own rewards.

◁ Generous kaphas are the world's best cooks and decorators, with large circles of friends. They make wonderful party hosts.

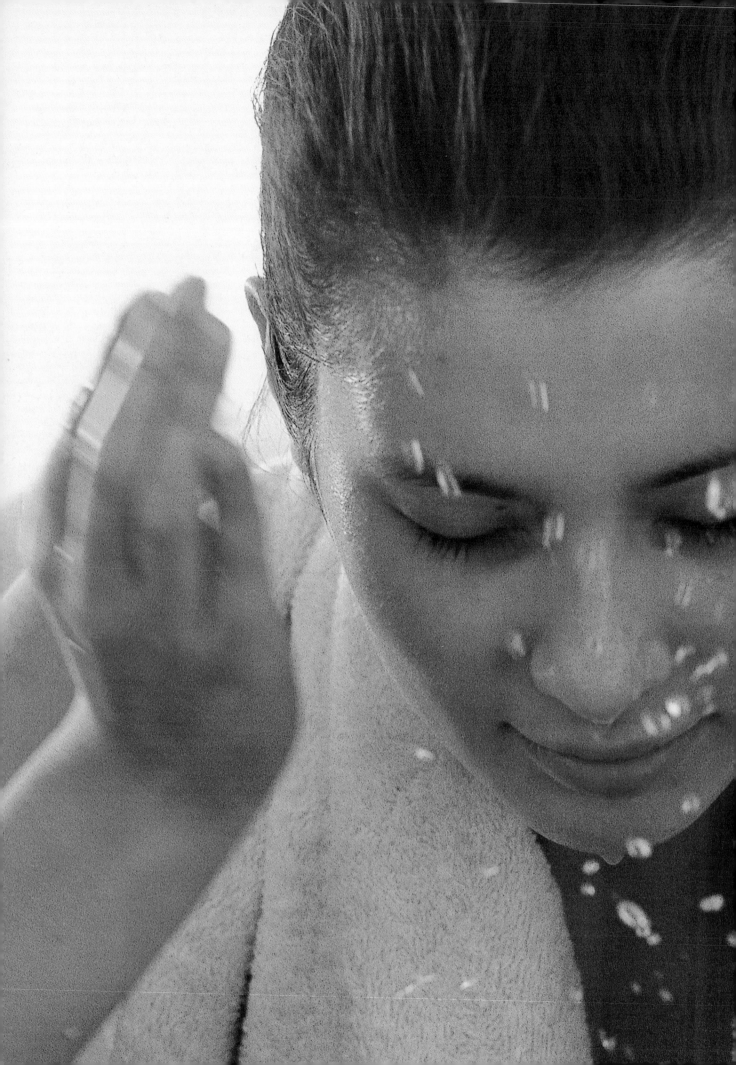

Cleansing the Body, Clearing the Mind

Ayurveda aims to promote natural beauty and lifelong

youthfulness by keeping all the systems in balance.

The first essential is to clear the systems of

anything that hinders this aim. In physical

terms, it includes cleansing treatments

such as massage, steam therapy and

fasting. For the mind and spirit it

means discarding old habits of

thought that clutter up

the consciousness.

Healing hands

Massage plays a central role in Ayurvedic treatments, stimulating circulation and promoting the elimination of waste. Different versions are used to treat illness, heal injuries, aid detoxification, calm the mind, beautify the skin and rejuvenate the body. These treatments can now be found at Ayurvedic centres worldwide.

Abhyanga is the classic full-body massage, carried out by one or two therapists. As well as stroking and kneading movements, the therapists apply finger or hand pressure to some of the body's 107 marma points.

Champissage is a specialized head massage that stimulates marma points across the head, aiming to tone up all the body's systems. It helps to improve circulation, boost the immune system and slow down the aging process.

Shirodhara consists of pouring warm oil slowly on to your forehead while a therapist massages it gently into your scalp.

Pottali or **Navrakhizi** is a massage with hot poultices of rice, oil, milk and herbs. The resulting paste is washed off and more oil is massaged in. Traditionally used to treat vata conditions, it's as beneficial for stress and anxiety as for bodily aches.

Sarvangadhara or **Pizhichil** requires three therapists. One keeps a constant supply of oil warmed while two others dip linen cloths into the oil and squeeze it over the entire body, massaging it in lightly. This is a rejuvenating treatment that also aims to build up the immune system.

oil essentials

In Ayurvedic practice, oil is believed to help clear toxic ama out of the body. It also reduces excess dosha, which is considered to stick like a solid substance until softened and flushed out in the form of bodily secretions. Oil should be washed off after a treatment, so any waste products released into it don't re-enter the body.

MASSAGE FOR YOUR DOSHA

All dosha types benefit from massage. Vata people, and others who have dry skin, should always use oil for massage. The pitta dosha can be over-stimulated if too much oil is used, so just enough should be applied to avoid dragging the skin. Any kind of massage helps to provide the stimulation a kapha body requires, but deep-tissue massage is especially useful in aiding waste disposal via the lymph system.

You can choose an oil purely because it is suitable for your skin type. But if you feel that you are suffering from an excess of one of your energies – light-headed vata, for example, or impatient pitta – choose an appropriate oil for your dosha. Take outside influences into account: if it's a damp evening in spring, for example, kapha energy will already be high.

Full body self-massage

Ayurveda recommends self-massage each morning. As you do it, vary your touch so that you're sometimes moving your hands lightly over the skin, and at other times pressing firmly enough to move the skin over the bone. Use the fingertips for static pressure, but the softer pads of the fingers for kneading or circling movements. Avoid putting pressure on any joints. Unless otherwise stated, any pressure should be upward, towards the head. Always warm the oil, and make sure the room is pleasantly warm. Start by pouring a little oil into one palm and rubbing your hands together. Repeat from time to time as the oil wears off your hands. If you prefer not to get oil in your hair, you can do the head massage without it.

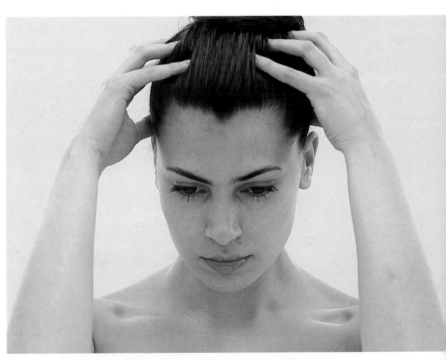

△ **1** Press your hands against your scalp and move the skin in large circles. Run your fingers through your hair and gently tug and rotate small sections of it to stimulate the scalp. With the tips of your fingers and thumbs, make little circles all over your head.

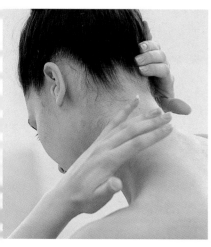

△ **2** Smooth oil into your neck and work it up over the back of your head. Cup the base of the skull in your palms and press gently upwards.

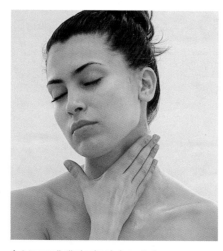

△ **3** Run well-oiled palms in long strokes up your throat from the collarbones, covering the front and the sides; repeat several times.

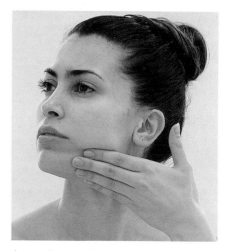

△ **4** Cupping your chin in each palm alternately, run the fingers up along the jawline to the ears several times, using firm pressure without dragging the skin.

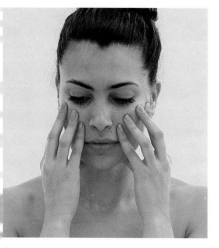

△ **5** Place your thumbs on your temples and massage the forehead in small circles with your fingertips. Use light pressure, and keep the movement upward and outward. Massage the cheeks in the same way.

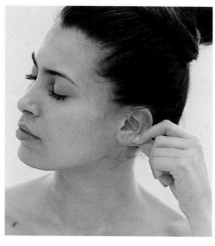

△ **6** Continue massaging in small circles all over the scalp and along the base of the skull. Gently pull and twist sections of the hair to stimulate the scalp. Then rub and squeeze the ears and massage all around them.

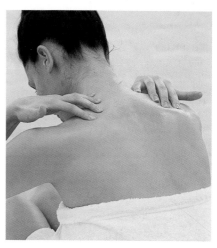

△ **7** Relax your head and shoulders and let your head sink forwards, keeping your shoulders down. Place your oiled palms on the back of your neck and rub firmly from the spine out to the sides.

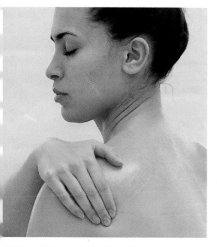

△ **8** Rub oil into each shoulder with large circular motions, using your whole palm and fingers. If you have any stiffness, cup your hand around the joint and rotate it as far as you find comfortable.

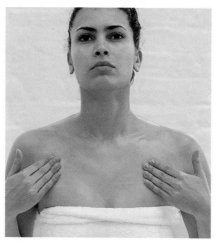

△ **9** Stroke oil outwards across your chest from your breastbone. Pull the fingers outwards in a semicircular movement, from the nipples towards the armpits, both above and below the breasts.

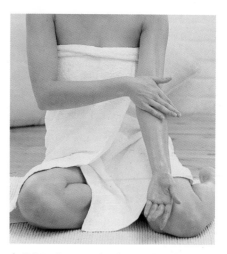

△ **10** Extend one arm, thumb upwards, and stroke lightly down the outside of the arm with your palm. Then reverse the movement and rub more firmly back up the inside of the arm.

continued over page ▷

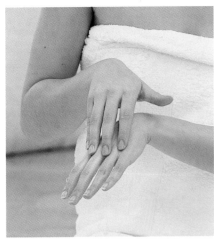

11 Grip your left arm just below the shoulder (▷), squeezing it between your fingers and the heel of your right hand. Move your hand a couple of fingers' width down your arm and repeat, working your way down to the hand. With the left hand extended, palm down, massage the wrist and the back of the hand (△) with the right hand. Grip and release the side of the wrist (▽). Repeat, working down the side of the hand to the fingertips.

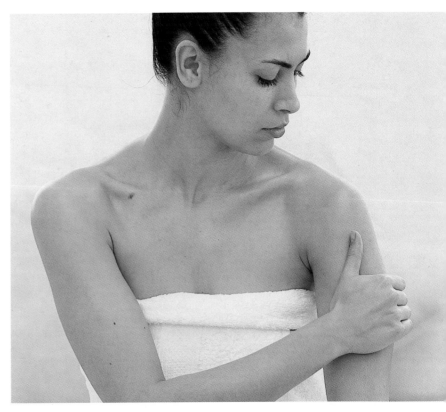

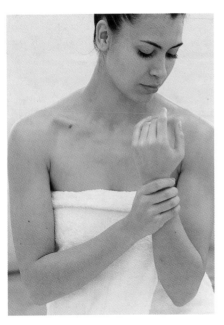

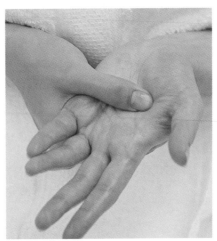

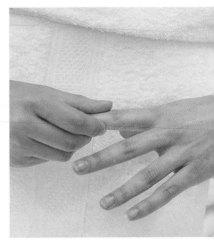

△ **12** Hold the left hand and massage the palm with your right thumb (above left). Now squeeze and massage each finger, finishing by pulling it gently (above right). Interlace your fingers and stretch the arms out in front of you, palms facing outwards. Keep your shoulders relaxed and low. Release your grip. Turning your left palm down, rub briskly up from the back of your hand to the shoulder. Repeat the arm and hand massage on the right.

CURING OIL

Oil for Ayurvedic massage is traditionally "cured" before use. To cure oil, pour it into an enamelled or non-metallic pan, add a drop of water and place over a gentle heat until the water pops, then remove from the stove. When cool, pour the oil into a glass bottle and store away from light. Just before a massage, warm a little of the oil to a comfortable temperature.

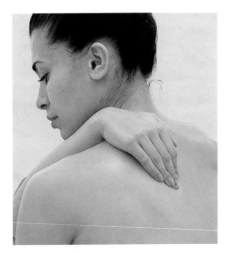

◁ **13** Reach over each shoulder with your fingers pointing downwards. Rub as far as you can stretch down and across your back, and press your fingers in as you pull back up, feeling that you are stretching the muscles upwards.

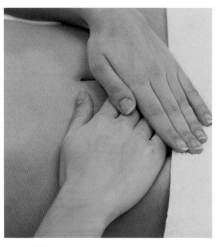

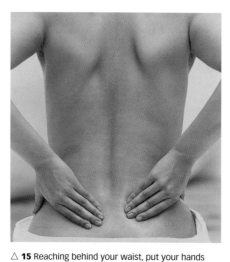

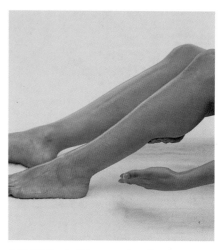

△ **14** With fingers pointing downwards, massage your abdomen with the flat of your hands in large clockwise movements, above and below the navel. If you suffer from poor digestion, you may massage with your fist, slowly circling down on the left and up on the right. Finish by stroking outwards from the centre.

△ **15** Reaching behind your waist, put your hands flat on your lower back, with fingertips on the spine, and draw them out to the sides, pressing firmly. Massage your hips and buttocks briskly with kneading, pummelling and large circular stroking movements, being careful to avoid direct pressure on your hip joints.

△ **16** Lightly rub oil down your legs, then massage up the calf muscles. Grip and release, or rub firmly in circles with fists spiralling upwards, or simply stroke firmly up towards the knees. If you have varicose or visible veins, stroke gently without any pressure.

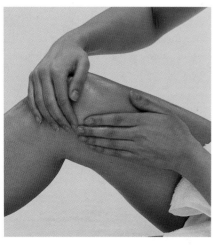

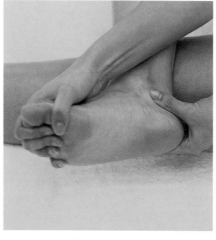

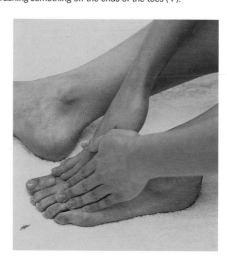

△ **17** Work gently over each knee, rubbing the kneecap, sides and back of the leg in circles using plenty of oil. Then stroke vigorously up the insides of the thighs, with brisk overlapping movements, into the groin.

18 Massage your feet one at a time. To begin, cup the heel in one hand and, with the other hand, grasp the toes and gently rotate the foot (△ above left) in both directions. Massage lightly over the ankle and top of the foot in circles, using more pressure on the sole to avoid tickling. Gently rotate each toe (△ above right). Finish by stroking firmly down from the ankle several times as if brushing something off the ends of the toes (▽).

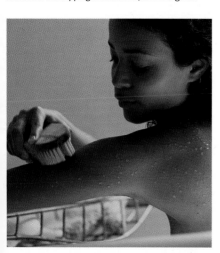

A TOUCH OF SILK

The full-body massage can be done without oil, using a glove made of raw silk instead. Pitta and kapha types should try this as a change from oil. Body-brushing, using a natural bristle brush or a textured mitt, also stimulates lymph circulation, which helps the body rid itself of waste products.

◁ **Use a natural bristle brush for a stimulating body massage while you are bathing.**

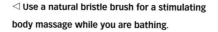

Painless detoxification

Spring is traditionally the time for detoxifying. *Swedana*, or sweat therapy, adds to the benefits of massage by helping the body cleanse itself through the pores, while a cleansing diet eases the pressure on digestion, promoting radiantly clear skin and boundless vitality.

steaming

For deep cleaning the skin, steam baths offer an easy solution and the benefits are instantly noticeable. The moist heat allows the pores to open and sweat flushes out impurities. Steam softens the outer layer of skin, encourages renewal by increasing circulation, and helps shed the dead cells – traditionally removed with a metal scraper. For those who can't stand damp heat, or who suffer from an excess of kapha dosha, a sauna may be an effective alternative.

Start with a shower, then oil your skin while still damp, before entering the steam room, to nourish the skin and bring your dosha back into balance. Shower again after steaming, and finish the treatment with a refreshing cool splash: the combination of hot steam and cold pool or shower is profoundly revitalizing.

At home, enjoy the benefits of steam by running a very hot bath and oiling your skin while you relax beside the bath and wait for it to cool. Throw a bag of herbs into the water, choosing a blend to suit your skin or your dosha. When the bath is a comfortable temperature, massage the oil off with an *ubtan*, or herbal powder, then bathe off the residues and finish with a cool shower.

a cleansing diet

Rigorous fasts can cause health problems, including a serious vata or pitta imbalance, but semi-fasting for a few days can help clear accumulated waste. Choose vegetables, fruits and grains that suit your dosha.

• Start the day by drinking a cup of hot water with a dash of fresh lemon juice, and add some honey if you wish.

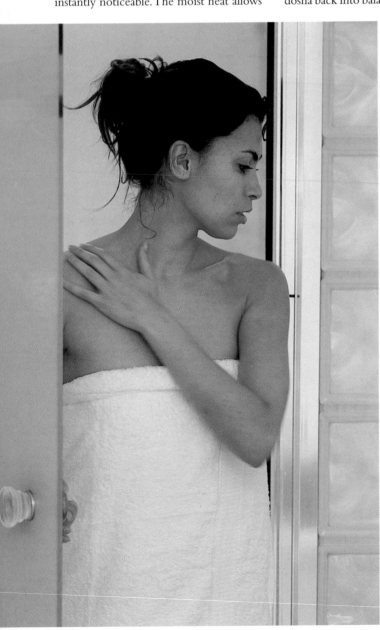

◁ **Oil your skin before a steam bath and shower afterwards, using a massage mitt or sponge to slough off dead skin and leave yourself glowing.**

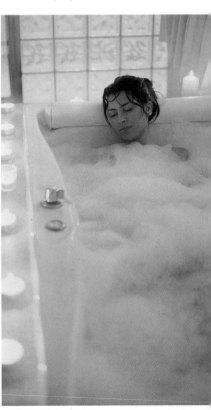

▷ **A bath offers two ways to benefit from the effects of hot water. Run it very hot and sit beside it, luxuriating in the steam. When it's cooled enough, step in and relax.**

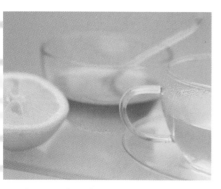

△ **Wake up to the refreshing taste of hot water with a splash of lemon and a trickle of honey.**

• For breakfast, at least half an hour later, squeeze some fresh fruit juice.
• A light lunch should be your main meal, consisting of boiled or steamed vegetables and grains. Eat slowly, so you notice when you're comfortably full.
• In the early evening, drink some fresh vegetable soup or vegetable juice.
• Throughout the day, except within about an hour of your lunch or supper, drink plain hot water or diluted vegetable juice whenever you wish.

If you're following this regime for less than four days, you can cut out the midday grains. Otherwise you can continue for up to 10 days, but no longer, because the diet does not provide all the nutrients you need in the long term.

the secret of eternal youth

Rasayana is Ayurveda's method of staying young. It includes taking herbal remedies selected by a practitioner, practising yoga asanas, and doing *pranayama*, or breathing exercises. Since toxins accelerate the aging process, it also means keeping your intake of these to a minimum.

Eating well becomes more than a question of balancing nutrients: food actually reduces your life force if it's stale, overprocessed, laden with chemicals or irradiated. Alcohol is doubly toxic, through its befuddling influence on the brain as well as its physical effects on the liver.

mental discipline

Ayurveda believes that your health and vitality are strongly influenced by factors such as the environment and your own outlook. Rasayana may require changing

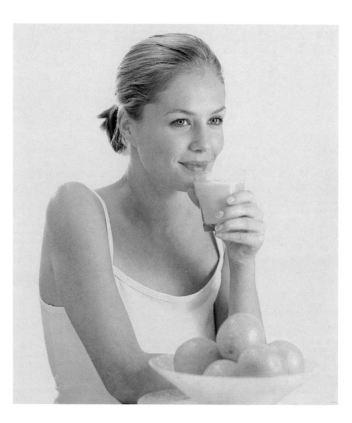

◁ **If you treat yourself to a juicer you can discover the full variety of vegetable and fruit tastes. Meanwhile, a lemon squeezer is all you need to turn citrus fruit into a delicious instant drink.**

your whole lifestyle. How much do you want to keep your energy and your wrinkle-free complexion?

You need to check whether you're producing toxic thoughts. Anger, envy, dishonesty, resentment, greed, callousness and even anxiety can all sap your life force. Just let such feelings go if you can; otherwise seek a practical short-term form of therapy to help root them out. If you spend too much time delving into the reasons for these unworthy thoughts, you're giving them undue attention.

What about your relations with the people around you? Ayurveda values harmony and teaches that you should seek to create it in all areas. If your efforts to free your mind of toxic thoughts are sabotaged by someone who drives you mad, either come to terms with them or keep out of the way. If it's a family member, listen to their grievances and try to understand them.

outside influences

Ensure that your environment isn't dragging you down. Bad air and water are obvious dangers. But do you live in an ugly environment? Can you often hear noisy neighbours or angry car drivers? If you're in the country, are you affected by chemical sprays? Are your surroundings more

demoralizing than invigorating? You can build up resistance to outside factors, but it all uses energy that could be better spent.

Your occupation and daily life should tend towards harmony, with the natural world as well as with other people. Is your job worth doing, or does it cause harm? Do you live a wasteful, high-consumption life? Consider whether you need to move house, change jobs or rethink your way of life.

▽ **Oiling the skin is an essential element of Indian beauty, and is also believed to help clear the body of ama, or toxic residues.**

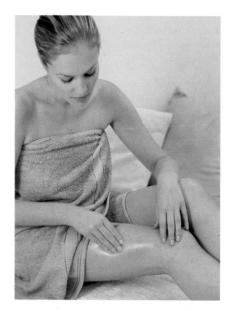

Bringing meditation into your life

The non-physical world is as real to Ayurveda as the one we can see and touch. Its elements, routes and effects are described in texts and on maps that are as detailed as an anatomy textbook. All the levels of existence constantly impinge on each other, and any toxin or blockage in one can harm another.

Meditation is part of the detoxifying process, clearing waste products from the mind, and is a central part of a beauty regime. By counteracting stress and promoting a balanced lifestyle, meditation brings tangible health benefits that show on your face and body. Among other ill-effects, depression can cause weight gain from comfort-eating; anxiety can cause facial lines from tension; a hectic lifestyle can cause skin disorders from indigestion.

Since the 1960s, meditation has become popular in the West, but it's still widely misunderstood. Meditation is not a magical process or a quick route to nirvana. It's simply a way of focusing the mind, freeing up mental energy that's usually wasted. It aims to still the mental chatter that runs endlessly through our heads, making work more difficult and relaxation impossible. Surrounded by noisy distractions and conflicting demands on our attention, we probably need meditation more now than ever. Even when we're engaged in something we enjoy, we're often only partly there, with the rest of our mind wandering off along other tracks. Meditating helps us to live in the moment.

CAUTION

In rare cases, meditation can trigger psychological problems. Go to your doctor if this happens, since the meditation may have revealed a disorder in need of treatment. Also check with your doctor before starting meditation if you have any medical condition, especially one that affects your heart or blood pressure.

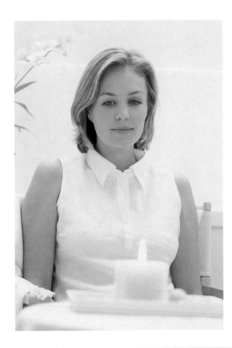

△ **A candle flame can be an aid to meditation – a simple, calming point on which to focus while your mind comes gently to rest.**

alpha waves

Each time you meditate successfully, your heart slows, your blood pressure drops and your brain starts to produce alpha waves instead of the usual beta waves. This relaxed but alert alpha state is distinct from day-dreaming, dreaming in your sleep or sleeping without dreams: your brain is producing quite different electrical activity.

You may have experienced the alpha state by chance, since it sometimes happens naturally when you are relaxing at the end of a yoga class, watching the sun set or listening to peaceful music. When you slip into it you feel a sense of deep contentment and niggling worries vanish from your mind. You may be startled to realize some time later that you had quite forgotten something

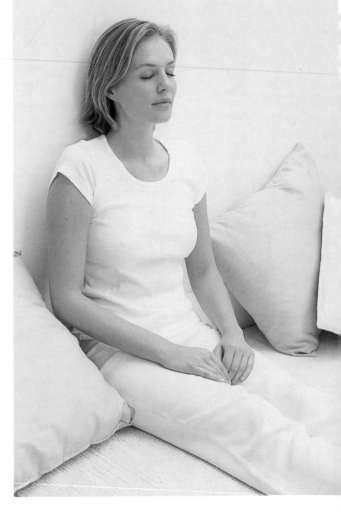

▷ **In the Western world, we feel we have to keep busy. Ayurveda, with its concept of balance in all things, reminds us of the value of stillness too.**

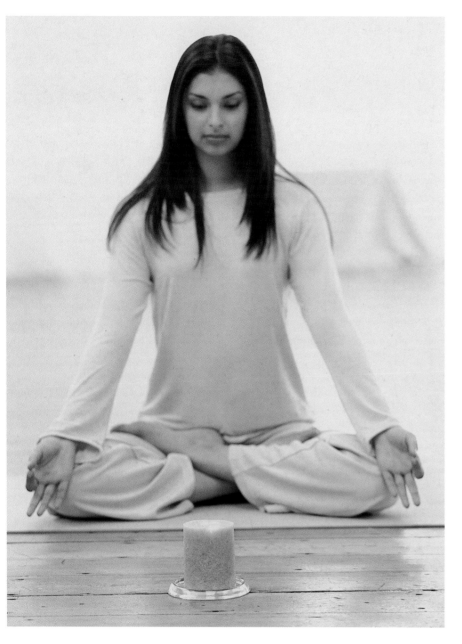

◁ **Most cultures have developed techniques to still the mind: another traditional method is prayer. Both individuals and society can benefit from rediscovering a peaceful space.**

how meditation can help

Medical science agrees with Ayurveda that meditation is good for you. As well as clearing your mind and aiding relaxation, meditation increases your powers of concentration, assists physical healing and slows the aging process.

Large-scale studies show that regular meditators have fewer illnesses and hospital admissions. Controlled trials have proved its benefits in many health conditions, not all of them traditionally linked with stress. These include cancer, migraines, irritable bowel syndrome, asthma, anxiety, mild depression, high blood pressure, heart disease and the degenerative processes of old age. One study, reported in *The Journal of Behavioral Medicine*, compared 423 practitioners of Transcendental Meditation with 1,757 other healthy adults and found that the meditators had levels of the age-related hormone DHEA-S similar to people 5–10 years younger. People with high DHEA-S levels are found to suffer less breast cancer, osteoporosis and cardiovascular disease.

▽ **Just one session of meditation can leave you feeling better, and long-term practice can transform your life.**

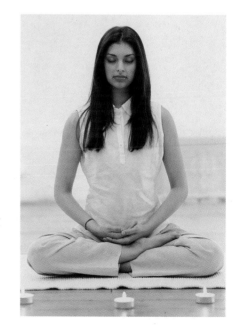

that was bothering you. Meditation is a simple technique for finding that calm space when you need it.

In beta state, you may have tried to concentrate on a task till your eyes crossed, but it's hard work. Let your concentration slip for a moment and the background chatter of your mind takes over. The skills practised in meditation make it easy to focus on what you're doing. Moving into alpha state almost at will, you can take a break before refocusing on what you were doing and completing it more easily.

learning to meditate

There are many different methods of meditation, and the choice is yours. The best-known form is Transcendental Meditation, or TM, established in India in 1957 by the Maharishi Mahesh Yogi, who subsequently introduced it to the West. This offers personal tuition, your own mantra (a word to repeat while meditating) and follow-up sessions to iron out any problems.

Devotees claim that the mantra given to them by a TM leader is more beneficial than one they could have made up for themselves, and even sceptics admit that they're more likely to persevere with something they've paid a week's wages to learn. If you've tried meditation by yourself before and found it impossible to establish a routine, TM could be the answer for you, but many people have done it for themselves, learning from books, on a one-day course or from a friend.

How to meditate

Meditation involves keeping your attention on something without being distracted. The conscious mind throws up a series of obstacles to this: your head is filled with mental chatter, you can't get comfortable, you have a brilliant idea, you've just remembered something important. As these distracting thoughts enter your mind, let them drift out again without giving them your attention. When, inevitably, you realize that your mind has wandered, calmly bring it back to the meditation.

It's easiest to get into the habit of meditating if you do it at the same time and place every day. It doesn't have to take long: set a timer for 10 minutes once a day and you may notice improvements before the end of the week. Start by doing a seated meditation, one of the most basic Ayurvedic forms. Sit on a comfortable straight-backed chair with your feet on the floor, and then close your eyes.

Whatever form of meditation you do, it's important to keep your breathing steady and remain aware of it. Pranayama – breath control – is one of the essential steps in the anti-aging therapy rasayana, and underlies successful meditation. Always keep your back straight to let energy move freely.

counting breaths

The simplest way to start meditating is to count your breaths. Let your breathing slow down, then count each breath just before you take a new one. Count up to 10, then start again. Keep your attention on your

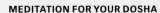

◁ **The basic meditation pose: sit with your spine comfortably straight – neither slumped nor stiff – and your feet flat on the floor. Closing your eyes helps bring you into a meditative state.**

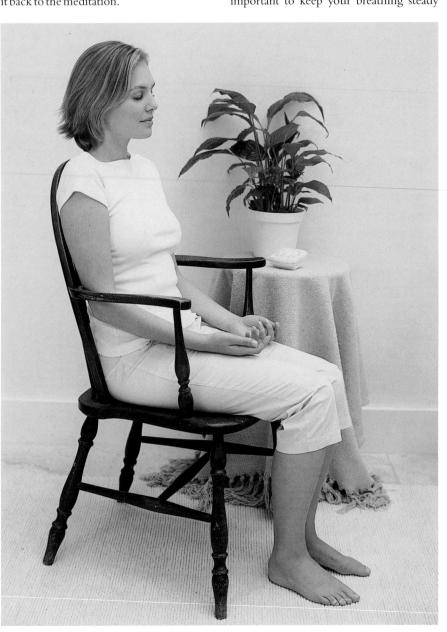

MEDITATION FOR YOUR DOSHA

Vata energy is speedy, so if this dominates you'll gain a lot from the calming effects of meditation. You'll probably find it hard to sit quietly for long, but you may be motivated by chanting or moving meditation. If your dosha is aggravated, choose a slow and calming method rather than, say, dancing. Try to practise some seated meditation, because this is a powerful calming and centring force.

Pitta dosha gives you the drive to succeed at whatever you take up, as long as you feel it's worth doing. You can benefit from all kinds of meditation, working on emptying your mind. As you try to clear the space, any obsessive thoughts soon make themselves obvious, but just waft them away. Mindfulness meditation is also ideal, giving you something else to occupy that space.

Kapha people are naturally quiet and calm, so you don't need to do a lot of work on stillness. Instead, try working on keeping the mind focused. Physical activity is always useful for kapha dosha, so you may get more benefit from a moving meditation. Try the livelier forms, such as dancing.

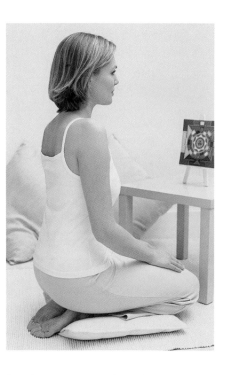

◁ **Many people find it easier to clear their mind of distractions when they have something to look at, such as the intricate patterns of a mandala.**

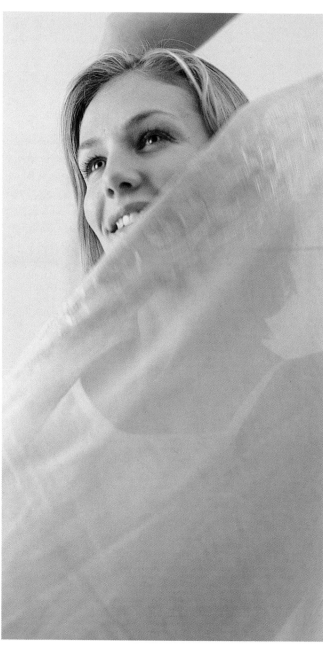

breathing. Note how the air feels as it enters and leaves your body. Before long your breathing becomes steady and it becomes easier to bring your focus back after each detour. You stop fidgeting and begin to feel a sense of peace.

mantra meditation

A classic form of Ayurvedic meditation is repeating a sacred sound, or mantra. Stay with it while the sound becomes irritating, then meaningless, simply keeping your attention on the sound. If you learn Transcendental Meditation you will be given a personal mantra. Otherwise, repeat a word or phrase such as "Om", "Peace", "Stillness" or "I am calm". If you use a real word, focus also on its meaning and try to feel nothing but that quality filling you.

mandala meditation

Gaze at one of these beautiful, complex figures and feel the devotion that went into creating it. Keep your focus on the mandala itself, letting any thoughts it inspires drift away. Let yourself blink naturally.

candle meditation

There's something immensely peaceful about gazing at a candle, making this ideal for times when you feel upset. Focus on the flame, without letting your imagination take over: just be in this moment. Remember to blink naturally.

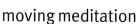

▷ **Let your spirit express itself with dance: the graceful swirl of movement will help to clear your mind of thought and let you slip into the alpha state.**

moving meditation

Some people find it easiest to reach a meditative state through movement, which prevents restlessness. Yoga, with its emphasis on breath awareness, is popular, and other meditative exercises such as t'ai chi are equally effective. A simple method is walking slowly, regulating your steps to the slow rhythm of your breath.

When you become experienced in this kind of meditation, you can bring the same focus of mind and awareness of breath to other activities that are just complex enough to engage your mind without effort, while remaining aware of your steady breathing. An exercise that involves rhythmic movement, such as swimming, is helpful.

Dancing can be wonderfully uplifting, as long as you do it without self-consciousness – even though your breathing speeds up, the music and joyful movement can flip you into the alpha state.

mindfulness

A different route to the alpha state is mindfulness meditation. Instead of trying to switch your mind off, focus fully on what you're doing. When you're massaging yourself, for example, be totally aware of the fragrance of the oil, the feel of your skin, the nurturing movements of your hands. As with all meditation, when you notice that your mind has wandered, just bring it gently back without criticism.

The colour of energy

According to Ayurvedic philosophy, colours have healing or harmful properties that can affect our bodies as well as our moods. Each shade contains different wavelengths of light energy, and generates different vibrations that subtly affect our own energies. The body's seven important energy centres, the chakras, are depicted in the form of many-petalled lotuses or whirling wheels of colour. These centres draw in energy from the universe and supply it to our physical and non-physical bodies. The energy channel that connects all the chakras follows the course of the spine.

using colour

The effect of colour is recognized by many people who don't care about the theories but just do what works: they paint fast-food eateries bright red – to make us eat up and leave quickly – and hospitals in healing blues and greens. We are acknowledging the power of colour when we see red, feel blue, lapse into a brown study or walk around under our own personal grey cloud.

Like everything else, shades of colour have *gunas*, or inner qualities. You can train your eye to pick out those that are sattvic: their clear tones promote harmony and

▷ **Green is an ideal colour to use for a workplace, as it balances *tejas* – the mental fire that fuels intellectual efforts – and promotes a feeling of calm alertness.**

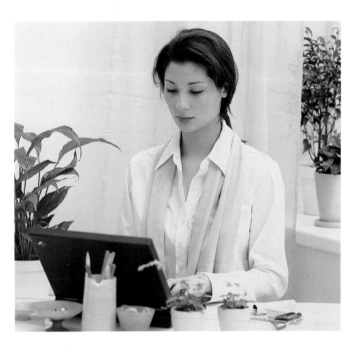

enlightenment. Harsh, over-bright rajasic hues put your nerves on edge, and muddy tamasic shades dull the senses.

Though we can't always control the colours that surround us, we can choose what to wear and how to decorate our

▽ **If you're run down or lethargic, surround yourself with energizing colours and feel them gently raise your spirits.**

homes. An insomniac whose bedroom is red or orange, for example, would be well advised to redecorate in a gentle shade of blue. If you sometimes feel out of touch with reality, repaint any white walls with warm pastels. Sombre colours (including certain cold shades of blue) can deepen depression. A clear violet will help you to pray or meditate, and green will keep your judgement unclouded while you work.

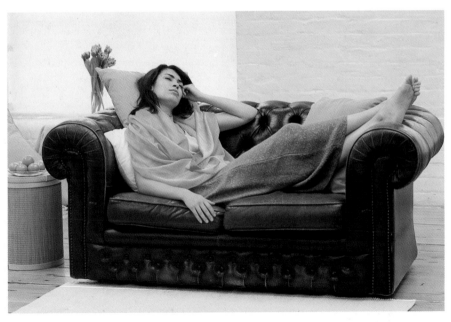

COLOURS FOR BALANCE

When your dominant dosha is aggravated, you can choose colours that help bring it back into balance.

Vata needs warming and grounding with colours such as red, orange or yellow. Avoid violet or purple, which can make vata types light-headed. Pastel shades such as pink are often helpful.

Pitta needs cooling colours such as blue, violet or white. Avoid red, orange, yellow, black, and rajasic shades of any colour.

Kapha needs warm, bright, energizing colours such as red, orange, yellow or violet. Avoid brown or grey.

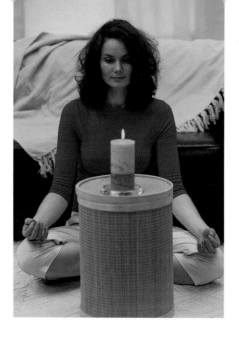

▷ Warm colours have a nourishing, grounding effect on light-headed vata, and can help create a state of relaxed alertness. These rich shades ease feelings of coldness and dryness.

the chakras

Ayurveda teaches that each chakra governs a different part of the body and supplies a distinctive kind of energy. A blockage in one of the chakras will cause specific diseases or emotional disorders. If you feel that you have a problem in one of these areas, try visualizing the chakra bathed in light of its own colour while meditating.

Muladhara, the root chakra: The first chakra is situated just behind the genitals. Its colour is red, and it is the source of strength and stability. The first chakra governs the body's eliminatory systems and its influence makes you practical and grounded. When it

is blocked or damaged in some way you may suffer from lower back pain, or become angry or disorganized.

Svadisthana, the sacral chakra: The second chakra is orange and lies just below the navel. It inspires passion, sexuality and creativity. It governs the reproductive system. Potential problems include sexual problems, self-pity and cystitis.

Manipura, the solar plexus chakra: The third chakra is yellow and provides willpower. It rules the digestive system and many internal organs. Problems include fear, low self-esteem and digestive disorders.

Anahata, the heart chakra: The fourth chakra is green and it is the source of compassion and equilibrium. Its area of influence is the heart and blood circulation. Problems include despair, unbalanced judgement, heart and lung disorders.

Vishudda, the throat chakra: The fifth chakra is blue. It rules the mouth and the thyroid gland, and the ability to learn. Problems include sore throats and difficulty in speaking out.

Ajna, the brow chakra: The sixth chakra, or third eye, is indigo. Situated in the middle of the forehead, it is the source of intuition and governs the nervous system and pituitary gland. It is the spot we instinctively touch when trying to think. Problems are nightmares, lack of concentration or detachment from reality.

Sahasrara, the crown chakra: The seventh chakra rules the pineal gland and is the source of enlightenment. It is shown coloured either violet or white – which contains all colours. If the crown chakra is blocked you may feel confused, or behave selfishly and unethically.

▽ Tranquil shades of blue and clean, clear white help keep pitta cool on even the hottest days.

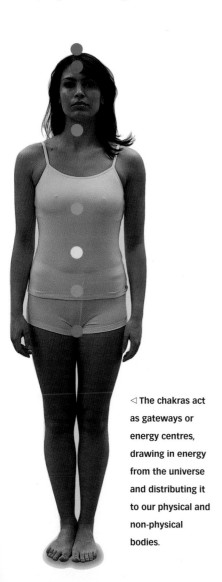

◁ The chakras act as gateways or energy centres, drawing in energy from the universe and distributing it to our physical and non-physical bodies.

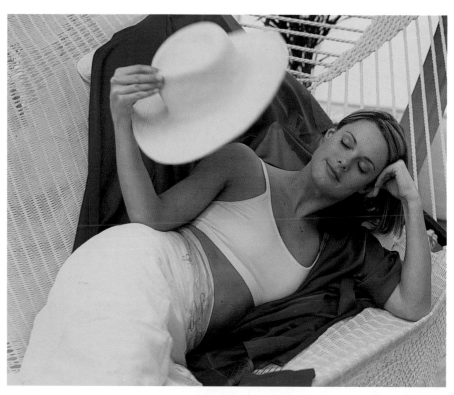

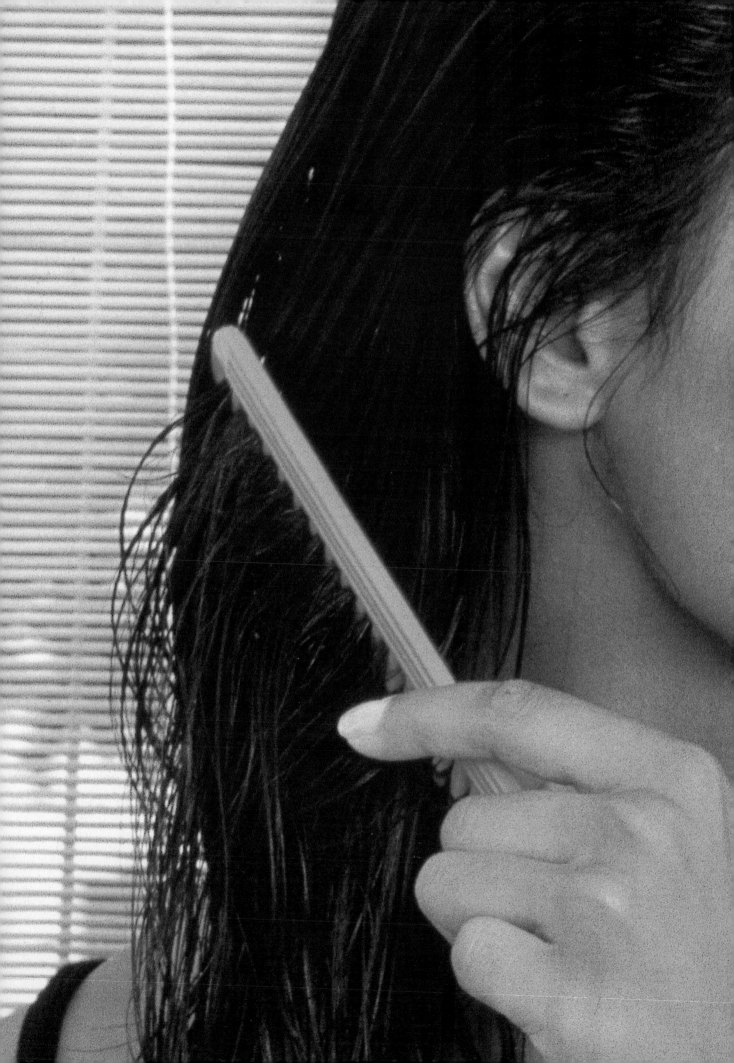

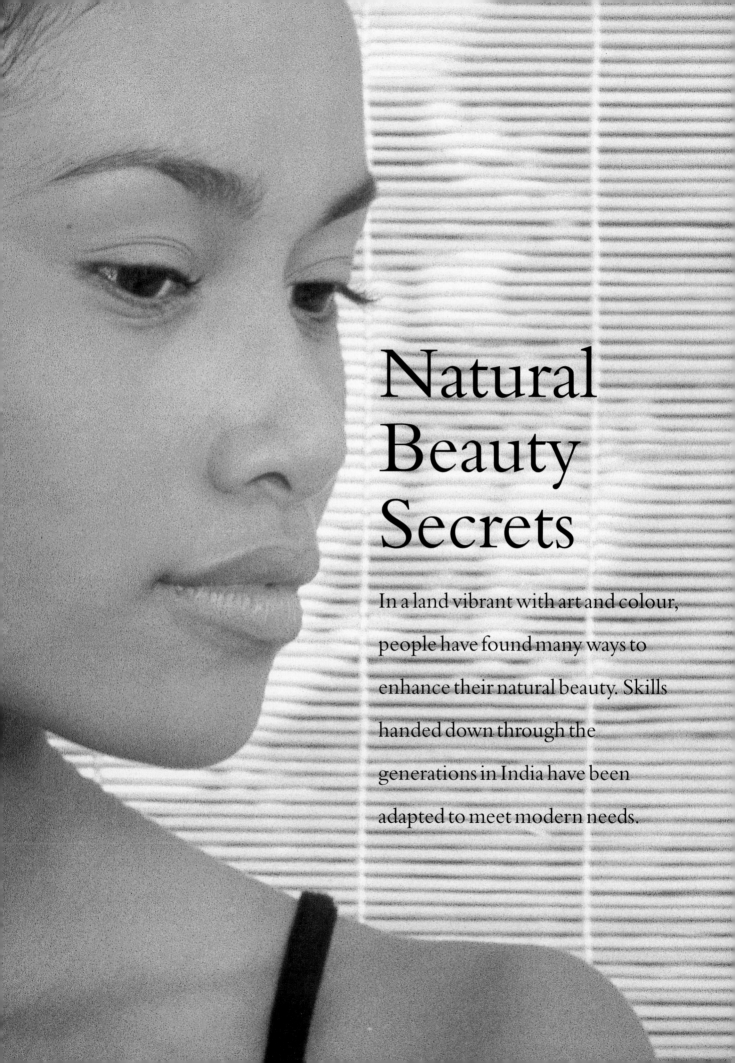

Natural Beauty Secrets

In a land vibrant with art and colour, people have found many ways to enhance their natural beauty. Skills handed down through the generations in India have been adapted to meet modern needs.

A home facial

Ayurvedic beauty treatments don't just improve skin quality: they're also an antidote to stress. The full routine for a facial treatment takes about an hour, so dedicate one evening every week or month to treat yourself luxuriously, but you can use the cleansing, toning and (for dry skins) moisturizing steps of this facial every day. Commercially made Ayurvedic beauty products are internationally available, but for those who like to make their own, recipes for each stage of the treatment are given on the following pages.

cleansing with oil

Oil is a good make-up remover for all skin types, and is ideal for cleansing off city grime or dust. You can make up your own blend, using a suitable base oil for your skin type, or use a base oil alone. Apply oil with your fingertips in a circular motion. Instead of washing the oil off, Indian women traditionally blot it up with a herbal powder called an *ubtan*.

ubtans

These powders clean and stimulate the skin, and can be used as a cleanser alone or after applying oil. The simplest ubtan is a mix of plain besan (chickpea or gram flour) made into a paste with a few drops of liquid: use lemon juice for oily skin or warm milk for dry skin. The paste should be firm and not too liquid. Apply to the skin with the fingertips using circular or upward movements, and when it feels dry massage it off with warm water.

More complex mixtures, containing herbs and grains, are used as exfoliants, usually after a herbal heat treatment. For skin that's not blemished or sensitive, it's a good idea to use a slightly coarser formulation every few weeks, always avoiding the delicate eye area. If your skin is sensitive, though, ensure the ubtan is finely ground – and resist that enthusiastic pitta tendency to scrub too hard.

▷ **Oil is excellent for removing make-up and nourishing all types of skin. It enters the finest pores without causing harm. Almond oil, rich in Vitamin E, is the traditional favourite.**

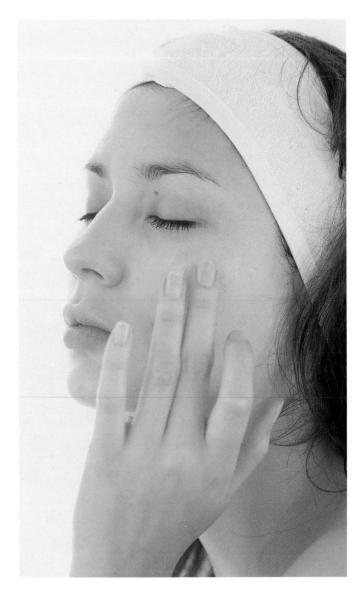

herbal heat treatment

A weekly heat treatment suits most skin types, though once a month is enough for dry and mature skins. Damp heat opens the pores, encourages sweat to flush out ingrained dirt and brings oxygen-rich blood to renew the skin. You may choose to put oil on your skin first, since the heat helps the oil penetrate more deeply. But don't leave cleansing oil on, or you'll be drawing dirt back into the skin.

Herbal steam: Sit with your head forward over a bowl of hot, herb-infused water, draped in a towel to stop the steam escaping, for about 5 minutes. Stop immediately if you feel dizzy or overheated.

Herbal compress: Soak several face cloths in hot, herb-infused water, and wring out. Sitting with your head back and supported, put the cloths over your face and relax for 5 minutes. As the cloths cool down, wring them out in the hot water again.

Herbal bath: Infuse a bag of herbs in your bath and let the heat open your pores.

Finish by patting your face with a clean cloth wrung out in cool water. Give your face a cooling splash of toner or water, then rest for a few minutes to cool down.

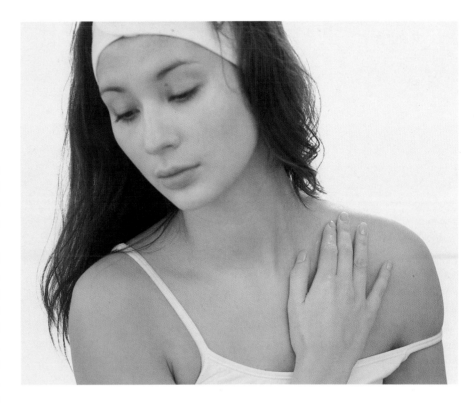

▷ Any nourishing or rejuvenating facial treatment, such as an oil massage, should work upwards from below your collarbones – an area that is all too often neglected.

oil massage

This is a traditional Indian technique. Oils are highly prized in Ayurveda, and considered essential to the healthy functioning of the body, but moisturizer can be used instead of oil if you prefer.

Warm some oil and pour a little into your hands. Starting just below your collarbones, smooth it into your skin using long strokes upwards and outwards, or clockwise circular movements. Continue for up to 10 minutes, covering your throat and face. Your touch should be just firm enough to move the skin slightly, without dragging it. Be especially careful not to drag dry or mature skin. Those with kapha skin should wipe off the oil before continuing.

facepack or mask

Few treatments give your skin such a quick lift as a facepack. These simple treatments, based on fruit or vegetables, can be left on for up to an hour, while you have a massage or meditate (you may need to be lying down if the mask is runny; try the Corpse yoga

▽ Take a break while the mask does its work – use the time for some other pampering treat.

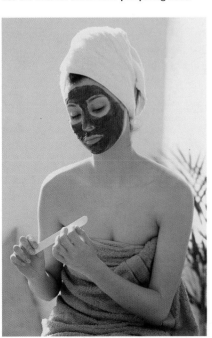

pose). A mask is a stronger version of a facepack, using a powder such as flour or clay to penetrate the pores more deeply. It should be left on for 10–20 minutes.

To remove the facepack or mask, dab it with water (for oily skin) or milk (for dry skin) to soften it, then gently massage and rinse the mix off your skin.

toning

Remove any residues and soothe the skin with a splash of cool flower water or, for oily skin, witch hazel and flower water. Skin that is very oily or has darker patches can be rubbed with a slice of lemon and left for a few minutes before rinsing off.

moisturizing

Only moisturize skin that feels dry. If you have oily skin or acne and follow the Ayurvedic process, you needn't use a moisturizer – none of the cleansing recipes will strip the skin of oil.

▽ A slice of lemon helps lighten darker patches, but don't use this on dry or sensitive skin.

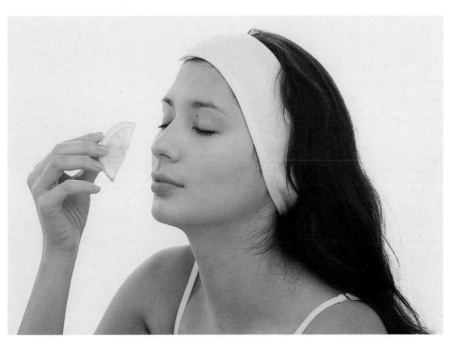

First step: cleansing

Traditional wisdom is a dynamic resource, adapting to new conditions as it passes down through the generations. Indian families who move to other countries often modify their age-old recipes to suit what they have to hand, replacing ingredients that are hard to find outside India with others that are easily obtainable, including essential oils.

You can turn your kitchen cupboard into a beauty treasure-trove, as practically all the ingredients needed for the following recipes are used in everyday Indian cookery. All are available from Asian stores, and most can be found in supermarkets.

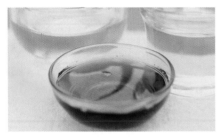

△ **Oils to suit your skin, from left: almond for all complexions, sesame for dry, sunflower for oily.**

cleansing cream

The best oils for cleansing are almond, sesame and sunflower. Alternatively, you can use this light cream cleanser.

ingredients

- 7.5 ml/¹/₂ tbsp beeswax
- 30 ml/2 tbsp coconut oil
- 30 ml/2 tbsp almond oil
- 60 ml/4 tbsp cucumber juice (or water)
- 1.5 ml/¹/₄ tsp borax
- 15 ml/1 tbsp witch hazel
- few drops rose water

ALLERGY ALERT

Before applying any cosmetic to your face, test it on your inner arm, leaving it for as long as you intend to leave it on your face. If any redness or irritation develops, wash off the mixture at once and discard it.

▷ **Ingredients for an ubtan (clockwise from front): ground coriander, liquorice sticks, besan, ground cumin and ground fenugreek.**

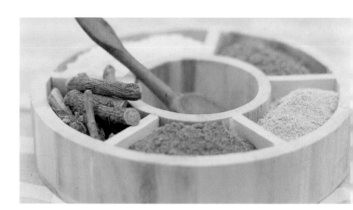

Melt the beeswax in a non-metallic bowl over a pan of hot water, and add the oils. In a separate bowl, heat the cucumber juice and borax (a good natural emulsifier) until the borax is completely dissolved. Add the witch hazel and remove from the heat. Combine the contents of the two bowls and allow to cool a little, then add the rose water. Beat the mixture until it cools and thickens.

herbal ubtan

This a traditional Indian cleanser. Many different blends are possible, but all have gentle softening and cleansing effects.

ingredients

- ground coriander
- ground cumin
- ground fenugreek
- ground liquorice
- besan (chickpea flour)

Mix together equal quantities of all of the ingredients and then store your mixed powder in a clean and airtight container. You will need about a small handful for one treatment. The dry base blend should be mixed to a paste consistency with the appropriate liquid ingredient for immediate use whenever it is needed.

- For oily, combination or blemished skin, mix the base blend to a paste with yogurt or diluted lemon juice.
- For dry or mature skin, mix the ubtan with milk or cream.
- For normal skin, or if the other combinations feel too sticky, mix with water or rose water.

Mix to a smooth, soft paste, then rub it into your skin – gently for dry vata or sensitive pitta complexions – using small circular movements. Massage off with warm, followed by cool, water.

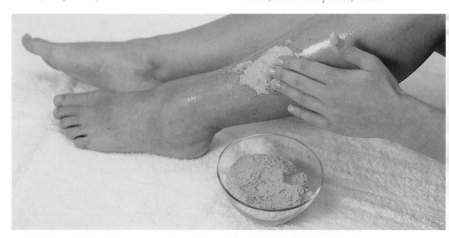

△ **If you've made more than you need for a facial, why not give your feet and legs a treat too?**

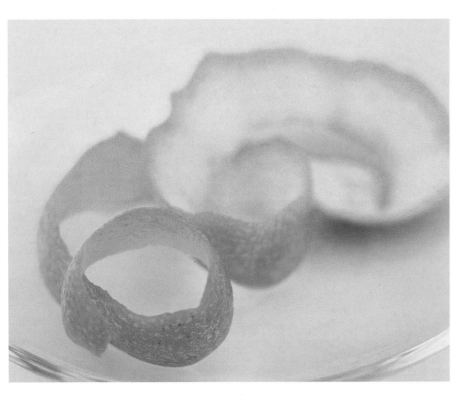

◁ Orange peel contains astringent oils that cleanse away excessive skin secretions and help to remove blemishes caused by blocked pores.

almond ubtan

This mixture is especially useful for reducing a pitta or vata imbalance, or for dry or sensitive skin.

ingredients
• walnuts
• fine oatmeal
• ground almonds

Grind the walnuts to a coarse powder and mix with equal quantities of the oatmeal and ground almonds. Store the mixture in an airtight container. To use, mix a small handful of the powder to a paste using water (for oily skin) or milk (for dry skin).

▽ Preparing ingredients, such as these walnuts for an ubtan for dry skin, is part of an almost meditative process of self-nourishment.

orange peel ubtan

This is useful for people with oily skin or a kapha imbalance, who should use it every second day. It helps remove blackheads gently and leaves skin feeling smooth. Start off by using equal quantities of all the ingredients. Later, you may decide to vary the proportions to suit your own skin.

ingredients
• lentils
• wheat
• dried orange peel
• fine oatmeal
• besan (chickpea flour)

Grind the lentils, wheat and dried orange peel to a coarse powder. For sensitive pitta skin, grind the powders more finely. Mix all the ingredients together and store the blend in an airtight container.

To use the ubtan, mix a small handful of the powder to a soft paste using a few drops of water, or lemon juice, or both, depending on your skin type. Use the paste as a facial scrub.

MILK AND SUGAR

These make the simplest facial. Moisten your face with water, then gently massage clean with a teaspoonful of sugar. Tone with a splash of water. Moisturize with skin from the top of boiled milk that's been left to cool. Leave this on for 2 minutes, then massage off with water.

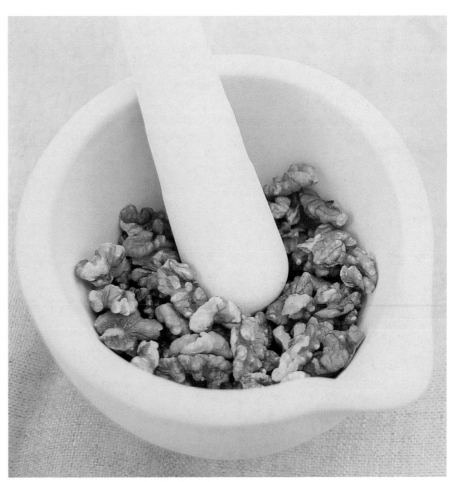

The next steps: heat and oil

For body massage, Ayurvedic practitioners normally choose an oil that will help to bring the doshas into balance, such as sesame oil to reduce vata or kapha and coconut oil to cool an excess of pitta. For the face and throat, however, they base their choice on skin type and condition – which are often an expression of dosha energy anyway.

In general, vata energy is expressed in dry skin, pitta in sensitive skin and kapha in oily skin. So you may wish to use treatments that suit your skin condition, while eating and following other guidelines to pacify the relevant dosha.

skin types

Classic vata skin is thin and fine-pored, dry, cool and often dark. This fragile complexion needs very gentle care and moisturizing. It should never be rubbed hard or dragged.

▽ For an easy steam treatment, pour a few drops of herbal oil blend into the bath and relax.

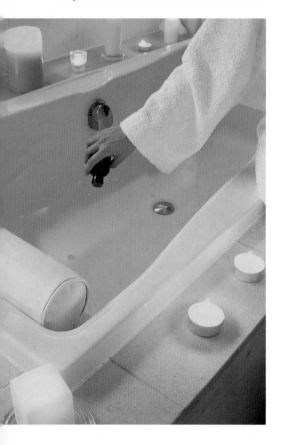

Pitta skin is soft, warm and rosy, but often sensitive. Avoid harsh chemicals or anything that could cause a rash or inflammation. Pittas often have combination skin, with an oily T-zone of forehead, nose and chin but drier skin on the cheeks and beside the mouth. Common problems are acne and patches of pigmentation.

Kapha skin is strong, thick and naturally moist. It's therefore slow to show signs of aging or environmental damage, but it is prone to enlarged pores, blackheads and excessive oiliness.

If, like most people, you are influenced by two doshas, you should note which one seems dominant in your complexion. You may be mainly kapha, but if your skin is sensitive to heat and chemicals, and is much drier on your cheeks and beside your mouth, it's expressing pitta energy and needs to be treated for this. Your skin condition will also vary with external factors such as the weather: the cold dryness of winter increases vata energy, for example, and may affect your skin accordingly.

herbal steam treatment

Add a scented mixture of herbs and spices to hot water for a gentle heat treatment. Test the steam with your inner arm before allowing it near your face.

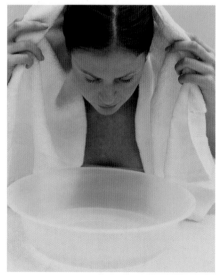

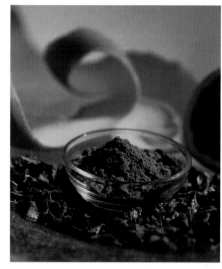

△ Fresh ingredients boiled in water release their fragrance and healing powers in steam.

ingredients
• half a lemon
• strips of orange peel
• pinch of pure sandalwood powder
• dried rose petals

Possible added ingredients you could use:
• For oily skin: liquorice root, lavender, fennel seeds, rosemary.
• For mature skin: liquorice root, fennel seeds, clove, grated ginger, mint.
• For dry skin: liquorice root, bay leaf, chamomile.
• For blemished skin: liquorice root, lemon grass, lavender, dandelion root.
• For normal skin: liquorice root, thyme, chamomile, fennel seeds, lavender.

Put at least 1.2 litres/2 pints/5 cups water in an enamelled or non-metallic pan and add the lemon and about two handfuls of a mixture of the remaining ingredients. Cover and bring to the boil, stirring occasionally, then remove from the heat. Leave covered and allow to cool until the steam is a comfortable temperature.

◁ If you're short of time – or herbs – even plain hot water can be used to steam oiled skin.

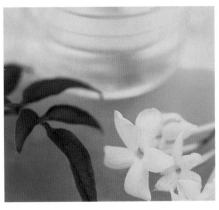

△ **Sesame or almond oil, infused with jasmine, makes a soothing massage oil for dry skin.**

facial massage oils

The base oils can be used alone, but do try making a herbal oil for face or body massage: two methods are given below. Some infused oils can be bought ready-made, or you could add a drop of essential oil. (A few essential oils should be avoided in pregnancy; check with an expert before using.)

simple herbal oil

ingredients

• handful of fresh herb (see box)
• 250 ml/8 fl oz/1 cup base oil (see box)

Crush the herb leaves using a pestle and mortar, then add a small amount of your

chosen base oil and blend thoroughly. Now add this blend to the rest of the oil, pour into a screw-top jar and shake well. Keep in a cool, dark place and shake several times a day for three days before using.

herbal oil infusion

ingredients

• 4 parts base oil (see box)
• 16 parts water
• 1 part ground or powdered herb (see box)

Measure the oil into an enamelled or non-metallic pan and add the water and your chosen herb. Bring to the boil over a medium heat, stirring briskly, then reduce the heat and leave to simmer gently, stirring occasionally, until all of the water has evaporated. Depending on the amount of infused oil you are making, this may take an hour or more. You could leave the pan on the back burner while you are preparing food, unless you are cooking something with a strong smell that could affect the oil.

▽ **Rosemary adds a clean, sharp tang to a herbal steam for oily or teenage skin.**

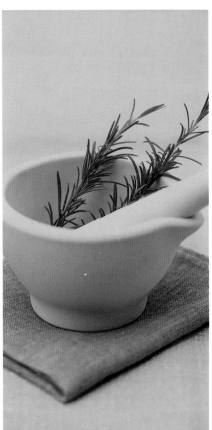

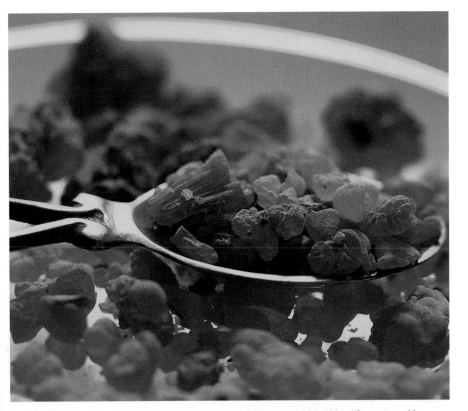

△ **So precious it was once a gift for kings, frankincense makes a nourishing blend for mature skin.**

Deep-cleansing facepacks and masks

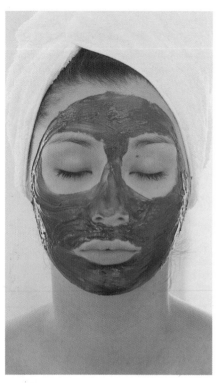

△ **Masks contain earth or flour, so don't apply near the delicate eye area or leave them on for more than 20 minutes, as they can be drying.**

Applying the very simplest cleansing and nourishing facepacks involves little more than squashing ripe fruit on to your face. Most fruits and vegetables can be used in this way, though harder types need to be grated or puréed: experiment with the suggestions given here to find what produces the best result on your skin. Smooth the facepack on with your fingers – or, if you find it easier, paint it on with a pastry brush kept for this purpose – and leave it on your face for up to 20 minutes (unless stated otherwise) while you relax. At the end of that time, massage the facepack off your skin and then finish by rinsing with water.

Clay, oatmeal or besan (chickpea or gram flour) can be added to any of the facepack recipes to make a mask that aids the cleansing process by drawing out dirt from deep in the pores. Oat flour is very soothing for eczema, while chickpea flour can leave skin feeling very taut, so is best combined with other dry ingredients. Mix the mask to a consistency that won't slide straight off your face – experiment on the back of your hand – and leave for up to 20 minutes before massaging and rinsing it off.

simple facepack

ingredients

• selection of fruit and/or vegetables (see box)
• 5 ml/1 tsp yogurt or almond oil

In a non-metallic bowl, chop, grate or mash the fruit and vegetables to a pulp. Strain off the excess juice for a healthy drink, and add the yogurt (for oily skin) or oil (for dry skin) to the pulp. Spread or brush the mixture over your face and neck, avoiding the delicate skin around the eyes. Lie down for at least 10 minutes while it takes effect, then massage and rinse off with cool water.

skin rejuvenator

This is kind to mature skin and can help reduce the appearance of wrinkles.

ingredients

• handful of fresh scented geranium (*Pelargonium graveolens*) leaves
• rose water to cover

Soak the geranium leaves in rose water for a few hours until softened, then spread on your face and lie down for 15–30 minutes.

avocado facepack

Egg white and lemon juice usually suit oily complexions, but the addition of avocado, rich in natural oils, makes this a great soother for dry skin too.

ingredients

• 1 avocado
• 5 ml/1 tsp lemon juice
• 1 egg white

Mash the avocado, mix in the other ingredients and apply to the face.

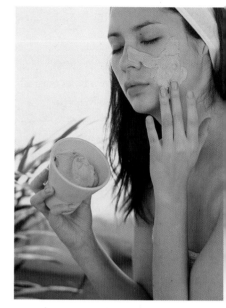

△ **Experiment to find what suits you: the richness of avocado makes a soothing facepack.**

apple facepack

This suits all skin types. If you have very oily skin, you may wish to use jojoba oil instead of almond.

FACEPACK INGREDIENTS FOR YOUR SKIN TYPE

Sharp-tasting fruits, such as grape, lemon, tomato or peach, should be combined with a more soothing, starchy fruit or vegetable, such as banana. Be careful if you include grape in a mixture, as it has a peeling effect on the skin; don't use it at all if your skin is dry or sensitive.

• Normal skin: avocado, banana, courgette, grape, peach.
• Dry skin: avocado, banana, carrot, melon, pear.
• Oily or combination skin: cabbage, cucumber, lemon, pear, strawberries, tomatoes, tangerine.
• Mature skin: apple, avocado, banana.
• Blemished skin: apple, cabbage, plums (boiled and allowed to cool), tomato.
• In hot weather: cucumber, strawberries.

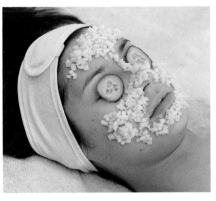

△ **Relax while an apple facepack rebalances your skin and cucumber reduces any puffiness.**

ingredients
- ¹/₂ small apple, peeled and grated
- 15 ml/1 tbsp honey
- 1 egg yolk
- 15 ml/1 tbsp cider or wine vinegar
- 45 ml/3 tbsp almond oil

Mix together all ingredients.

spot remedy facepack
ingredients
- 1 egg white
- 5 ml/1 tsp honey
- 5 ml/1 tsp carrot juice
- 5 ml/1 tsp crushed garlic

Beat the egg white until stiff. Mix in the other ingredients and apply for 20 minutes to help heal spots and blemishes.

honey and egg facepack
This instantly rejuvenates dry skin.

ingredients
- 2.5 ml/¹/₂ tsp honey
- 1 egg yolk
- 15 ml/1 tbsp dried skimmed milk

Mix to a paste and leave on for 20 minutes.

juicy mask
Yogurt cleanses the skin, while the juices feed it with vitamins and minerals.

ingredients
- 15 ml/1 tbsp powdered brewer's yeast
- 2.5 ml/¹/₂ tsp yogurt
- 5 ml/1 tsp orange juice
- 5 ml/1 tsp carrot juice
- 5 ml/1 tsp almond oil

Mix all the ingredients into a paste. If you have oily skin or darker patches, add 5 ml/1 tsp lemon juice; for very dry skin, double the oil content.

clarifying mask
ingredients
- 10 ml/2 tsp ground almonds
- 5 ml/1 tsp rose water
- 2.5 ml/¹/₂ tsp honey

Mix into a paste and apply as a thin layer. Rinse off with cool rose water.

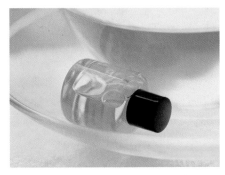

△ **Add a little light oil, such as almond or jojoba, to counteract the drying effect of face masks on delicate vata skin.**

oatmeal mask
Use yogurt to bind the dry ingredients if you have oily skin, or almond oil for dry skin. For other skin types, choose whichever you prefer – try one version on each cheek and see which feels better.

ingredients
- 10 ml/2 tsp fine oatmeal
- 30 ml/2 tbsp powdered orange peel
- yogurt or almond oil

Mix the oatmeal and powdered orange peel together and add enough yogurt or almond oil to make a paste.

potato mask
Rich in Vitamin C, potatoes also tighten the skin, making this a good choice for tired or mature complexions.

ingredients
- 15 ml/1 tbsp potato juice
- 15 ml/1 tbsp multani mitti (fuller's earth)

Mix together thoroughly to make a paste and spread on the skin.

BESAN (CHICKPEA FLOUR) MASKS
- For oily skin: mix besan with some olive oil and lemon juice.
- For dry or normal skin: mix besan with some olive oil and yogurt.

spot remedy mask
This is effective against spots and blemishes.

ingredients
- 1 egg yolk
- 15 ml/1 tbsp powdered brewer's yeast
- 15 ml/1 tbsp sunflower oil

Mix to a paste and apply to the face. After 15 minutes rinse off with milk.

orange mask
This is suitable for dry skin.

ingredients
- 5 ml/1 tsp freshly squeezed orange juice
- 15 ml/1 tbsp multani mitti (fuller's earth)
- 15 ml/1 tbsp rose water
- 15 ml/1 tbsp liquid honey

Mix all the ingredients together to make a paste and smooth lightly on to the skin.

EGG ON YOUR FACE
When you need to look good and haven't time for a full treatment, just try an egg. For oily skin, beat an egg white and spread on to your face. Leave to dry and then wash off thoroughly. This tightens skin for a temporary face-lifting effect. If you have dry skin, use the whole egg, beaten. You can also use egg white or whole egg, depending on your skin type, as a substitute for oil or yogurt in herbal ubtans and facepacks.

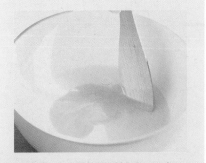

△ **Egg feeds the skin and binds powders.**

Finishing touches: toning and moisturizing

A splash of cool filtered or spring water refreshes skin after any treatment. Flower waters add their own natural benefits, and gently close pores without the harshness of alcohol-based toners. For oily skin, try water with a dash of vinegar, or rose water with a dash of witch hazel.

flower waters

Rose water is perfect for skin care. Mildly astringent, it soothes and rehydrates skin. It's cooling in a hot climate, reduces inflammation, and the subtle fragrance is said to have antidepressant and aphrodisiac qualities. Buy the highest quality you can find, or make your own.

Rose water makes a refreshing spray, especially in the dryness of air-conditioned rooms or the stuffy heat of a plane, and also helps to set make-up. A cloth or cotton pads wrung out in rose water and placed over closed eyes is the kindest treatment when your eyes are sore.

Other flowers can be used in the same way. Lavender water has long been prized for its cleansing, deodorant properties and refreshing scent. In hot weather it is ideal to use over the entire body – and also for spraying on clothes and bedlinen.

▽ **Simple pleasure: a splash of plain water revitalizes your mind and refreshes your skin.**

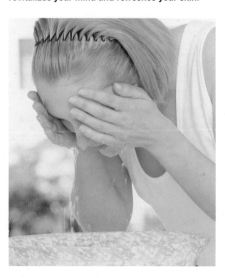

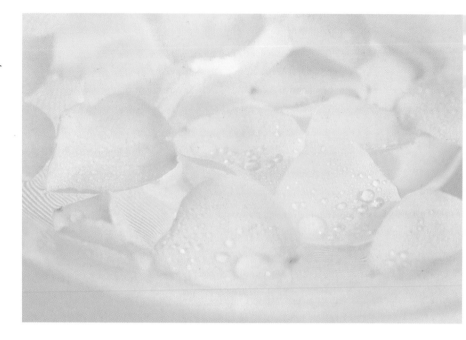

rose water

Use equal quantities, by volume, of rose petals and pure water to give a delicately scented result. Increase the water's strength by using more petals, as long as the water still covers them. For an even stronger scent, use dried rose petals: simply shake fresh petals into a paper bag, loosely close the top, hang up and leave to dry.

ingredients
- 1 cup fresh scented rose petals, tightly packed
- 1 cup spring or filtered water

Put the petals in a heatproof, non-metallic container. Boil the water and pour it over the petals. Cover and leave to cool. Decant into a screwtop bottle or jar and store in the fridge.

rose water astringent

For oily or blemished skin.

ingredients
- 1 part rose water
- 1 part witch hazel

Pour both ingredients into a screwtop jar or bottle and shake to mix.

△ **The fragrance of rose water has been treasured throughout history.**

rose water soother

A treat for a dry complexion and tired skin under the eyes.

ingredients
- 250 ml/8 fl oz/1 cup rose water
- 1 drop sandalwood oil
- 1 drop rose, tea rose or rose geranium essential oil

Pour all ingredients into a screwtop jar or bottle and shake to mix.

lavender water
ingredients
- handful of fresh lavender heads, stems removed
- 475 ml/16 fl oz/2 cups filtered or spring water

Put the flowers into a jar with a screw top and pour the water over them. Leave for a day, shaking occasionally. For a stronger scent, leave it for up to three weeks, taking the top off every few days to check the scent. Strain off the water into a clean jar or bottle and keep in the refrigerator.

flower water refresher

ingredients

- 1 part water
- 1 part rose water or lavender water
- 2 slices cucumber
- few drops lemon juice (optional, for oily skin)

Combine the water and flower water and refrigerate for 5 minutes. Dip the cucumber slices in the liquid and put over closed eyes while you rest. Pour the remaining liquid into a spray bottle, adding a few drops of lemon juice if you have oily skin. Use as a refreshing spritz for face and throat.

moisturizing cream

Adjust the measurements given to find a consistency that suits your skin, and choose a herbal powder to balance your dosha: white sandalwood or jasmine for pitta, manjishtha for vata, or neem for kapha.

ingredients

- 30 ml/2 tbsp beeswax
- 175 ml/6 fl oz/³/₄ cup almond oil
- pinch of herbal powder (see above) or a few drops rose or jasmine essential oil

Melt the beeswax gently in a non–metallic bowl over hot water. Stir in the oil. Add the herbal powder or essential oil, and whisk until the mixture is soft. Allow to cool.

▷ **For a subtle and unique fragrance, look around your garden and pick your favourite blooms to create flower water recipes of your own.**

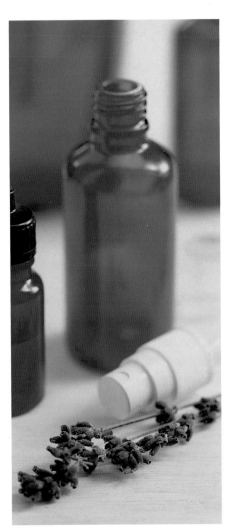

TAKE CARE OF YOURSELF

Don't hurry while giving yourself a facial. If time is short, it's better to leave out some of the steps than to rush through them. As far as possible, ensure that your surroundings are quiet and you're not interrupted. The results can be seen as stress dissolves from your face.

Preparation, too, should be a meditative process. Focus, one by one, on the colours of the ingredients, their textures as they are mixed together, the different scents as they develop, the small sounds of the spoon against the bowl and the feel of the various mixtures on your skin.

◁ **Keep some screwtop jars for mixing and spray bottles for spritzing. Remember to store all natural cosmetics – and even bottled water, once it's opened – in the refrigerator for safety.**

SAFE STORAGE

Traditionally, women grew their own plants or bought them freshly picked. They ground their own spices, grains and other powders, and used them immediately, whether in cooking or on their skin. Not many of us have a chance to do the same now, so we need to store ingredients safely.

Dry ingredients should be kept in clean, airtight containers. Stored in a dark cupboard, they should keep their fragrance and potency for weeks or months. Anything moist should be refrigerated to prevent the growth of moulds or bacteria. Since home-made cosmetics don't contain strong preservatives, mix them as you need them and don't keep the leftovers for more than a few days.

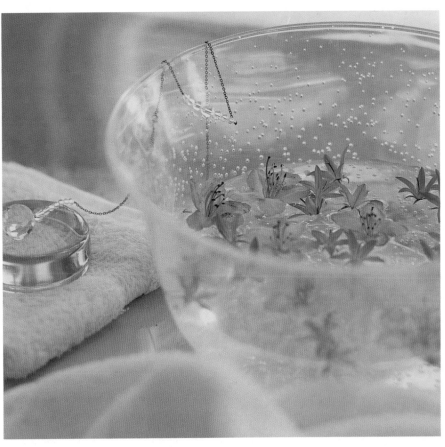

An Ayurvedic *facelift*

Your skin type, build and dosha will determine whether lines or sagging will be more of a problem as your skin ages. Generally, if you're thin and have dry skin you're more likely to develop wrinkles, a problem that besets many vata people. Kaphas are more likely to have oily skin and put on weight. This can bring beauty benefits, but the downside is that extra flesh starts to sag, causing a jowly effect. Anyone ruled by pitta or (like most of us) by more than one dosha could encounter any of these problems. So the best treatment aims to keep them all at bay.

Marma-point facial massage

A 30-minute daily marma-point massage will slow down the effects of time on your face. In Ayurvedic terms you're encouraging the movement of prana, the life force; Western science explains it as releasing muscle stiffness and increasing blood circulation. Sit with your back straight but not arched. It's useful to have a table to lean your elbows on, and to use a mirror to check the positions of your fingers, but close your eyes when you don't need to look. Before starting, massage your shoulders, neck and head for a few minutes: tension in these neighbouring muscles creates tension in your face.

VARYING PRESSURE

Throughout the massage you can either continue the 7–5–7–5–7–5 pressure used in step 1, or simply press once for a count of 7. Either way, press slowly and firmly, pressing inwards against the bone, not upwards or downwards unless specified. You can also vary the direct touch with small circling movements, maintaining the pressure and moving the skin over the bone.

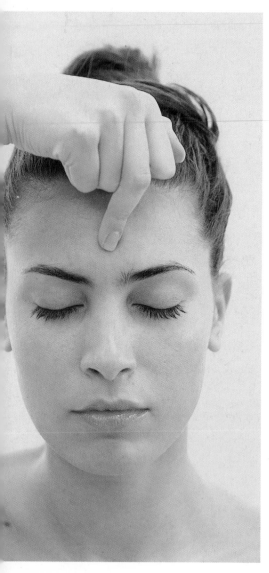

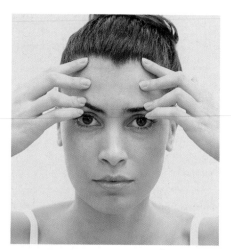

◁ **1** Begin by working on the Third Eye point, slightly above the bridge of your nose. Feel for a slight indentation, which is often the sign of an important marma point. Apply firm pressure for a count of 7 as you breathe out, then reduce to light pressure for 5, breathing in. Repeat 3 times.

◁ **2** Find the point in each eyebrow directly above the centre of the eye, and visualize a line from there up into your hair. Following this line, press your ring finger into the eyebrow point, the index finger into the hairline, and the middle finger between them.

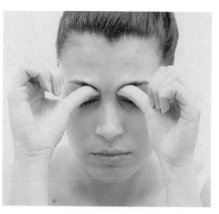

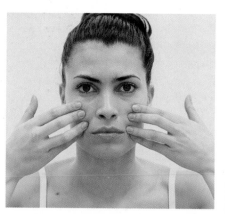

△ **3** Feel for the upper edges of the eye sockets and press firmly with the thumbs. Be careful to press the bone, without letting your thumbs slip into your eyes or eye sockets. Lift your thumbs, move them just above the eye sockets and press again, pushing upwards so that your forehead furrows.

△ **4** Place the tips of your index fingers on your cheek bones, with your other fingertips vertically below them under the centre of each eye, and apply firm pressure.

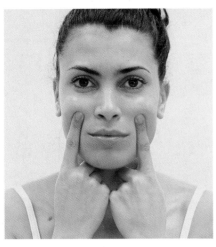

△ **5** Find a point directly below each cheekbone, still in line with the centre of your eyes. Press inwards and upwards into the bottom of the cheekbone.

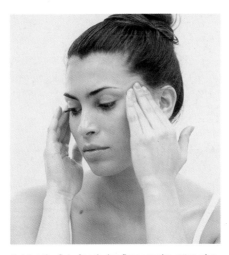

△ **6** Put the flat of each ring finger on the outer edge of each eye socket, and spread the other fingers out along a diagonal line to the edge of the ear. Press the fingers firmly.

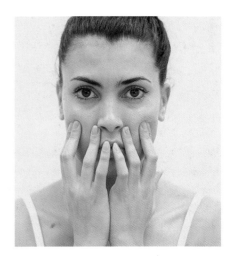

△ **7** Find a point at the outer edge of each nostril and press diagonally inwards with your third fingers, while your index and middle fingers press inwards and upwards below the cheekbones.

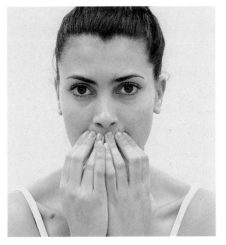

△ **8** Bunch all fingertips close together and press along the space between your top lip and your nose – an area containing numerous marma points. Do the same below your lower lip.

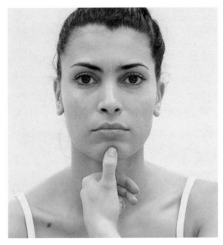

△ **9** Press one thumbtip into the centre of your chin.

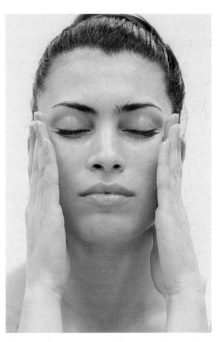

△ **10** If you like, pour a little oil or cream suitable for your skin type onto your hands. Bring your hands down the centre of your face, barely touching it, until the heels of your hands are under your chin. Now lightly stroke your fingertips out to the side across the cheekbones, without rubbing the fine skin directly beneath the eyes. Then bring the hands, with a firmer stroke, up the sides of the face. Repeat two or three times. Cup your hands over your closed eyes for several breaths.

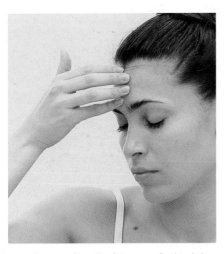

△ **11** Place your fingertips flat on your forehead, then stroke lightly towards the right ear. Repeat on the left. Stroke in both directions several times. If there's any feeling of drag, apply more oil to your skin. Continue the movement into your hair.

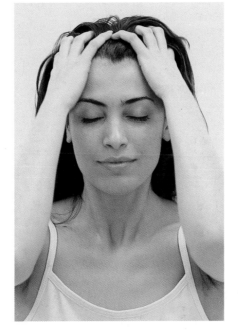

◁**12** Massage your head. Lightly pull sections of hair, making your scalp move in circles over your skull. Finish by combing with your fingers in long movements to the ends of the hair.

Body care

When you see the difference a facepack makes to your complexion, why stop there? Indian women have long enjoyed the benefits of herbal pastes, using them to enhance skin quality over the entire body.

Herbal baths are the easiest skincare treatment of all. Simply relax in a warm bath and let the ingredients nourish your skin while the heat eases away tension. Liquid ingredients can be poured straight into the water. Put other ingredients in a muslin bag, swish it around in the bath and leave it in while you soak.

body mask for oily or blemished skin

This mask is designed to detoxify, balance, remove impurities and polish the skin surface, leaving it silky smooth.

ingredients
- 115 g/4 oz/1 cup besan (chickpea flour)
- 5–10 ml/1–2 tsp turmeric
- 30 ml/2 tbsp white sandalwood powder
- 15 ml/1 tbsp red sandalwood powder
- 30 ml/2 tbsp neem leaf powder
- 30 ml/2 tbsp powdered orange peel
- water
- yogurt (optional)

Mix all the dry ingredients together and add water, or a combination of water and yogurt, to make a thin paste. Brush over the skin and leave for about 30 minutes, until dry. Wet the mask with water or milk, then massage off with fairly firm pressure. Rinse with water.

body mask for dry skin

ingredients
- 115 g/4 oz/1 cup besan (chickpea flour)
- 15 ml/1 tbsp white sandalwood powder
- 15 ml/1 tbsp red sandalwood powder
- 15 ml/1 tbsp Indian madder
- 15 ml/1 tbsp arjuna
- 15 ml/1 tbsp brahmi
- 15 ml/1 tbsp shatavari
- unhomogenized milk to mix

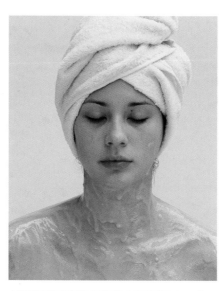

△ **Treat your whole body to a revitalizing mask that sloughs off dead cells, letting skin shine.**

Mix the dry ingredients then add the milk, warmed to body temperature, to make a paste. Brush this on to the skin and leave until it is dry. Remove with more of the warm milk.

bridal body mask

This is traditionally used by brides-to-be every day for 10 days before the wedding. It leaves the skin feeling soft and clean. A very simple form can be made using just turmeric and oil.

ingredients
- 15 ml/1 tbsp powdered orange peel
- 15 ml/1 tbsp powdered lemon peel
- 30 ml/2 tbsp ground almonds
- pinch of salt
- 25 g/1 oz/4 tbsp finely ground wheatgerm
- 15 ml/1 tbsp ground thyme
- 7.5 ml/1/2 tbsp turmeric
- almond oil to mix
- few drops jasmine or rose essential oil

Mix all the dry ingredients and add enough almond oil to make a paste. Add the jasmine or rose oil. Spread over the body and leave for 15–20 minutes. Rub off firmly, as though you are gently "sanding" the skin.

soothing bath mix

Add to the bath water to calm irritated skin, but don't use this on broken skin.

ingredients
- 120 ml/4 fl oz/1/2 cup cider or wine vinegar
- 30 ml/2 tbsp honey
- 120 ml/4 fl oz/1/2 cup lemon juice
  (or 115 g/4 oz/1 cup oatmeal)

If the sensitivity is intense, leave out the lemon juice as it will sting, and substitute a muslin bag of oatmeal.

▽ **A bath treatment to soften your skin can be as simple as a bagful of plain oatmeal swirled in the water.**

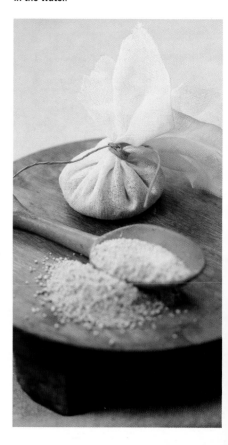

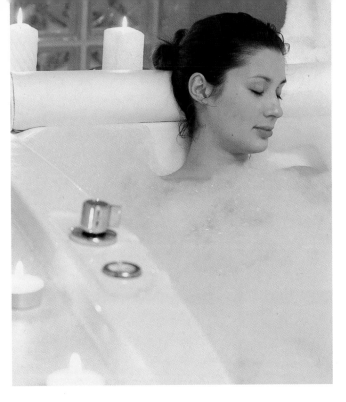

▷ Having your eyebrows professionally threaded gives long-lasting shape and definition, and you can learn to do it yourself.

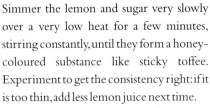

◁ Time to relax and let the tension drift out of tired muscles. Finishing with a cool shower gives skin a healthy glow.

skin softening bath mix

A very nourishing, soothing combination.

ingredients

- 45 ml/3 tbsp oatmeal
- 15 ml/1 tbsp bran
- 15 ml/1 tbsp ground almonds
- 15 ml/1 tbsp wheat flour
- few drops rose water

Put all the dry ingredients together into a muslin bag and add to the bathwater with the rose water.

milk bath

The classic: just add a few handfuls of powdered milk to the warm water and bathe like Cleopatra.

breast oil

Use this massage blend to tone and firm the breasts: the mustard oil makes the skin softer, while the powdered pomegranate rind has a firming effect.

ingredients

- 4 parts mustard oil
- 1 part dried pomegranate rind

Grind the pomegranate rind to a powder. Warm the mustard oil in a bowl over a pan of hot water. Mix the ingredients and leave to cool. Use the blend to massage the breasts with upward, circular motions, working outward from the nipples. Leave the oil on for at least 20 minutes, then rinse off with warm water and finish by splashing your breasts with cold water.

nail care

Whenever you're using oil, take a moment to rub some of it into your nails. Vata types often have pale, irregular nails that break easily. Pitta is linked with pink, oval nails that may be quite soft. Kapha nails are square and strong. All types can benefit from a hand cream of almond oil and honey.

hair removal

Women across Asia remove unwanted hair using the technique called threading. They hold one end of a cotton thread between their teeth, making a loop to lasso each hair, and tweak it out. This can be done professionally by beauty therapists. Easier to learn, and suitable for larger areas, is sugaring, using a mixture that is traditionally made at home. This can be made in large batches and kept in a jar. Sit the jar in hot water to soften it before use. It should last for a few months, as lemon is a natural preservative. You'll also need some strips of thick cotton, about 5–7.5 cm/2–3 in wide and 25 cm/10 in long.

ingredients

- 50 g/2 oz/4 tbsp sugar
- 30 ml/2 tbsp lemon juice

Simmer the lemon and sugar very slowly over a very low heat for a few minutes, stirring constantly, until they form a honey-coloured substance like sticky toffee. Experiment to get the consistency right: if it is too thin, add less lemon juice next time.

Allow to cool a little, then patch test to see if the temperature is tolerable. While still warm, spread on to the skin using a spatula. Place a cotton strip on the sugared area, press it down so that the warmth of your hands helps it to stick, and then pull off. On soft areas such as the calf, hold the muscle taut to prevent bruising.

▽ Practice makes perfect with sugaring, but the reward for your patience is silky smooth skin.

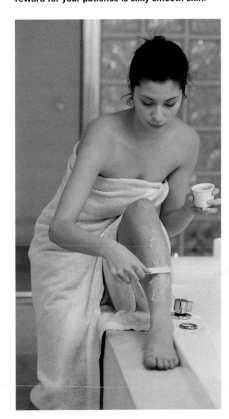

Gilded lilies: sparkling make-up

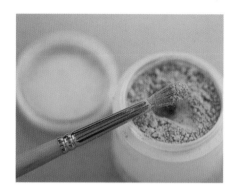

◁ **The warm shimmer of gold powder evokes the richness of India's beauty traditions.**

Gold has always been considered to have purifying qualities in Ayurvedic lore. Now it's being used to create pure cosmetics with a truly Indian sparkle. These dazzling innovations simply extend a long tradition of improving on nature's gifts. Make-up in India has been an art form for many centuries. Traditionally, emphasis was placed on the hair and eyes, but the hands and feet were also beautified with ornate henna designs and jewellery.

the traditional art

Everyone – men, women and children – wore cosmetics inside their lower eyelids. The intention was to prevent infection, as well as to make eyes look larger. Mascara-like blends such as kohl, kajal and surma were the most frequently used. The effect was exotic, and it remains popular today. A smear of castor oil made the eyelashes grow long and lush. Lips could be made to glisten with oil or ghee, and were given a deeper colour with crushed rose petals.

Even for those who could afford to wear gold jewellery, gold as a cosmetic colour was out of reach: only the members of royal families had the right to dust their skin with precious saffron, giving themselves a golden glow. Ordinary people might protect their skin with a light dusting of white sandalwood powder; red sandalwood powder brought fresh colour to pale cheeks. Overall, though, there was little emphasis on cosmetics for the skin, since this was meant simply to glow with good health. Most of the traditional preparations for skin were cleansers, toners and moisturizers – all aimed at improving the natural beauty of the complexion. Skin-covering preparations, such as foundation, were not widely used.

▽ **Natural ingredients are blended into cosmetics to enhance the healthy radiance of clear skin.**

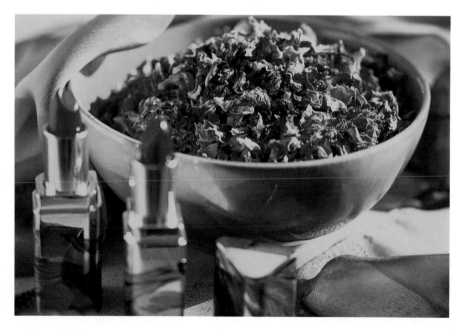

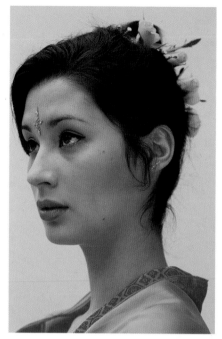

△ **Flowers, symbolizing life and happiness, are worn in appreciation of these blessings and to complement simple or sophisticated styles.**

new Ayurvedic cosmetics

Today's followers of Ayurveda have every kind of make-up at their fingertips – and they're using it to shine. Made from flower extracts, herbal essences and oils, modern cosmetic ranges aim to bring Ayurvedic beauty into the 21st century while retaining traditional holistic principles. Several companies offer protective foundations and sunscreens, incorporating natural ingredients such as clarified butter, honey, beeswax, kokum fat and jojoba oil. Some use antiseptic extracts from the neem tree as a natural preservative.

Ayurvedic rejuvenating treatments employ 24-carat gold leaf to give mature skins a youthful lift. In some cosmetic ranges it's included in blends of herbal extracts and spices that can be mixed with moisturizer to use as a foundation, giving a subtle sheen for the evening. Silver is also used in cosmetics, blended with herbs such as lavender to soothe pitta-reddened complexions with its cooling qualities.

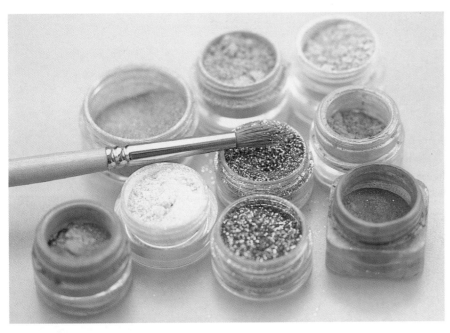

◁ A dazzling range of colours can enrich, conceal or emphasize features and create an individual palette. The lightest touch of shimmering powder draws attention to sensuous contours.

lip gloss

ingredients
- 15 ml/1 tbsp grated beeswax
- 15 ml/1 tbsp almond oil
- 5 ml/1 tsp honey
- few drops rose water

Melt the beeswax gently in a non-metallic bowl set over a pan of hot water, then stir in the other ingredients. Pour into a small pot with a lid and leave to set. Keep in a cool place. Apply with a finger.

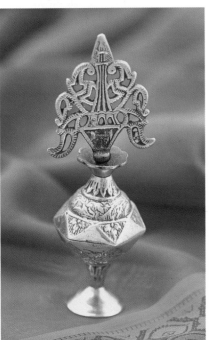

◁ Cool, clean silver is the metal of choice in which to preserve traditional eye make-up such as kajal.

traditional kajal

Place a clean spoon across the flame of a *diya* (a cotton-wick lantern burning ghee) and leave it there for a few hours to collect carbon from the smoke. Stay close by to avoid any accidents. Scoop the carbon into a clean ceramic container and mix to a paste with a little mustard oil. Apply with a fingertip, or roll the paste into a ball on the end of a slender rod, the size of a matchstick with the end whittled down.

▷ Nine centuries ago, the court poet Bilhana was willing to go to his death for daring to declare his love for "the gold-tinted king's daughter".

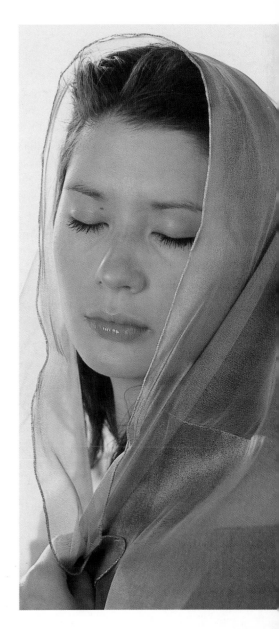

EYES RIGHT

The original Ayurvedic texts describe making kajal from a decoction of roots, berries, honey and the classic herbal mix triphala. Many women made their own version, using the soot from oil lamps mixed with camphor and oil or ghee. Pure kajal is soft, and was traditionally kept in a box made of silver, a metal considered to keep the contents cool and therefore soothing to the eyes.

Kajal is now sold around the world in many formulations, including pencils. But safety tests regularly expose kajal products containing dangerous levels of lead. Read the ingredients list, and use only products that have been certified to meet modern safety standards. Be careful too, as kajal can block tear ducts, causing temporary blurring of vision.

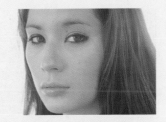

△ Kajal can be used to create strikingly beautiful "lotus eyes".

Shimmering tresses

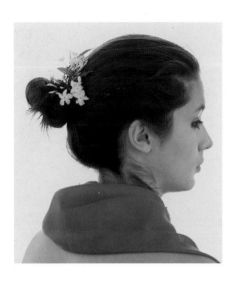

◁ **The fragrance of jasmine and its delicate, waxy flowers complement the gleam of sleek, shining hair.**

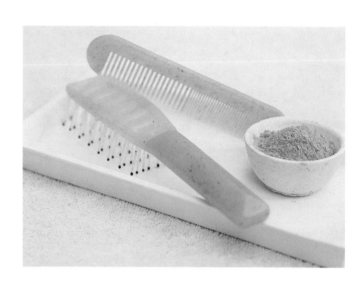

△ **Neem has many healing properties, and is available in the form of powder, oil or leaves. It has long been used to improve hair condition.**

Historically, perhaps no part of a woman's body has aroused more adulation than her hair. Throughout the ages flowing tresses have been praised in poetry and celebrated in art. In some cultures hair is still hidden to avoid tempting men or angels. The fifth-century Sanskrit poet Bhartrhari described a woman's hair as a forest, enticing the explorer into unknown territory where love waits like a bandit to ambush him.

Indian women have always been proud of their shining hair. The ancient carvings of Mohenjo-Daro and Harappa show women with their hair magnificently styled and jewelled. Traders carried perfumes from one continent to another for noblewomen to scent their tresses, jewellers created gold clips to hold their hair in place, and village carvers made combs of wood or bone for themselves and their daughters.

Lustrous hair is one beauty available to most women. The rich anointed their heads with priceless unguents and twined strings of gems through their artfully arranged curls. But any woman can scent and enhance her hair with a simple flower-sprig.

hair treatments

Traditionally, people massaged their hair with oil to keep it healthy and counteract the drying effects of heat. Fragments of a dried tree resin called sambraani would be burned and the hair allowed to dry in its fragrant smoke after washing. Harsh shampoos and chemical treatments were unknown. Despite the range of hair products now available, many people are turning back to tried and tested formulas, some of which blend traditional knowledge with modern convenience. Instead of crushing leaves from the neem tree to enhance hair condition, for example, you can now pick up a bottle of neem shampoo or conditioner.

Hair and scalp problems may suggest a dosha imbalance, though they may also be

▽ **Use your fingers to comb the mixture through your hair down to the tips before rinsing out.**

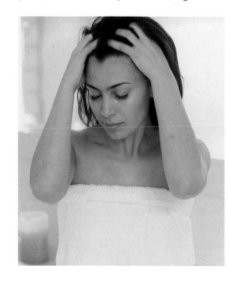

aggravated by stress, harsh shampoos, excessive heating or air conditioning. Dandruff, with a dry and flaky scalp, is frequently caused by the drying effects of aggravated vata dosha. But if the hair is dull and the scalp red and inflamed, the imbalance is more likely to be pitta – which is the commonest cause of hair problems. An Ayurvedic practitioner may suggest herbal remedies and massage with particular oils to calm the aggravated dosha. Changes to the diet are likely to include more green leafy vegetables, salads, milk, fruits and sprouts, buttermilk, yeast, wheat germ, soy beans, whole grains and nuts.

blends to combat dandruff

These blends can be made in a screwtop glass jar and shaken to mix before using. The mixture should be worked into the scalp and left on overnight if possible; if not, wait at least 3 hours before washing your hair.

• 5 ml/1 tsp camphor added to 120 ml/4 fl oz/½ cup neem oil.

• 5 ml/1 tsp each castor oil, mustard oil and coconut oil.

• 1 part fresh lemon juice added to 2 parts coconut oil.

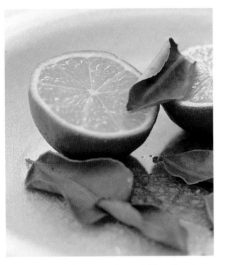

△ Lime juice helps to soothe an irritated scalp and leaves hair with a lustrous shine.

blends to soothe an itchy scalp

• 5 ml/1 tsp camphor added to 120 ml/ 4 fl oz/^{1}/$_2$ cup coconut oil. Massage the mixture into the scalp. Leave for at least three hours before washing off.

• Dried jasmine root, ground into a bowl of lime juice. Wash the hair and scalp with this mixture and rinse with lukewarm water.

rinses to add shine to the hair

• Squeeze a little lemon juice into a bowl of warm water and use as a final rinse.

• Add a little lime juice to a cup of rose water, add a cup or two of warm water and use as a final rinse.

egg conditioner

For dry hair, massage a beaten egg into the hair after washing and rinsing. Rinse out thoroughly.

rinse to prevent hair loss

Boil some neem leaves in water and leave to cool before straining off.

hot-weather conditioner

ingredients

• 1 egg
• 30 ml/2 tbsp castor oil
• 5 ml/1 tsp cider vinegar or wine vinegar
• 5 ml/1 tsp glycerine

To bring limp hair to life, mix the ingredients and beat well. Massage into the hair, leave as long as you like and wash out.

WHAT IS YOUR HAIR TYPE?

Like the rest of our bodies, our hair can show signs of our predominant doshas. If you're a dual-dosha person, you may feel that your hair seems to be out of line with your personality. How can a calm kapha have such dry, brittle hair? The answer is that your hair is reflecting your vata side while your inner self reflects kapha.

• If your constitution is mainly vata, you're likely to have dark, dry, coarse or frizzy hair that's prone to tangling, split ends and dandruff.

• Pittas are often blondes or redheads. They have enviable hair – fine and silky – but it needs looking after to prevent a tendency to go thin and grey before its time. It tends to be oily, but harsh shampoos make matters worse and can accelerate aging.

• People of kapha constitution may complain about their oiliness, but they have the least to worry about with hair that's naturally thick, glossy and wavy.

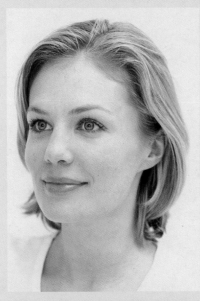

△ Pitta hair rewards gentle treatment with silky sleekness. Don't be tempted to use harsh products that may cause thinning.

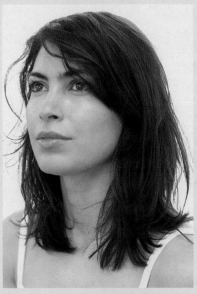

△ Kapha's fabulous mane grows long and thick at any age. If it shakes off efforts to control it, just revel in its exuberance.

▷ The traditional oil-based hair treatments used in India are particularly valuable for vata's dry hair, which is prone to tangling and splitting.

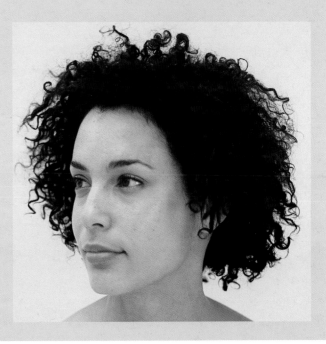

Enriching oil treatments

Traditionally, Indian women regularly treat their hair with oil, using vigorous circular motions of the palms and fingertips to work it well into the scalp and down the length of the hair. They leave the oil in until they next wash their hair and then oil the hair again as soon as it dries. It's an intense massage treatment that stimulates the scalp as well as coating the hair shaft.

The lustrous, gleaming effect used to be admired in Western countries too. These days, we tend to prefer a just-washed look, replacing the hair's natural oils with conditioner. But for a change, why not try a pre-wash oil massage instead? After the massage, wrap a towel round your head, and leave it on for a few hours or overnight. You may need to vary the amount of shampoo you use. Why not also try leaving off conditioner for a while, to see whether you really need it?

warming and cooling oils

Oil is used to strengthen and nourish all kinds of hair, but like most Ayurvedic treatments it should be tailored to suit the person. Your choice should also be influenced by external conditions such as the weather or the time of year. Coconut oil is popular for head massage, as it is renowned for its nourishing and strengthening powers. But it also has a cooling effect, which means it's best used in hot weather. The same goes for oil infused with brahmi – a valuable herb that's believed to stimulate the brain as well as the body.

In the winter, use a warming oil such as mustard or olive. Mustard is very nourishing and has a strong heating effect, though it smells rather strong. Almond is more neutral but has a slightly warming effect.

Choosing the right oil for the time of year is part of the Ayurvedic rhythm. But if you're feeling out of sorts, your need to balance your dosha by using particular oils may override this consideration. If you use a cooling oil in winter, stay in a warm room and don't go out till you've showered the oil off and dried your hair. If you use a warming oil in hot weather, rest until you feel more comfortable with the temperature.

hair oil and your dosha

Vata's typically dry hair will revel in the luxury of black sesame oil, showing its benefits in a rich lustre. Pitta needs very gentle massage with brahmi oil or coconut oil, to stimulate the scalp without damaging the follicles. These two oils are good for all hair types.

If you're kapha, good hair is your birthright and the only thing that's likely to go wrong is an excess of oil – possibly because you scrub your scalp too vigorously or use harsh shampoos. Use sesame or mustard oil, but leave it on for only 30–60 minutes before showering it off. Avoid stimulating the scalp with intense massage or when washing your hair.

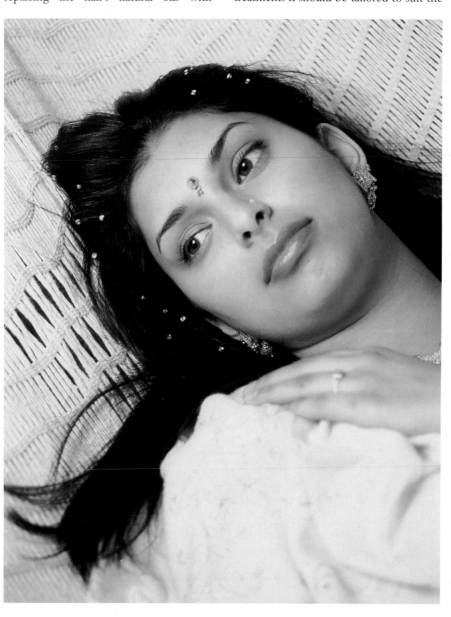

◁ **Luxuriant hair seems to come naturally to Indian women, whatever their dosha. Use of oil is one of their most effective beauty secrets.**

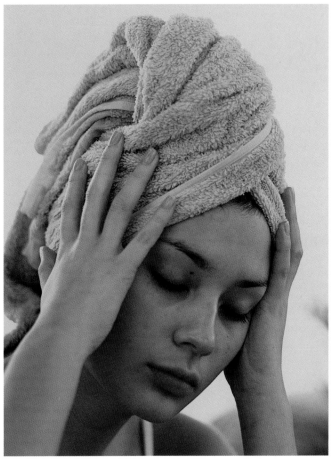

◁ **If you don't want to leave oil on your hair for long, wrap your head in a warm, damp towel after applying it, in order to aid penetration.**

warmth and penetration

Warming the oil before you use it on your hair can help it penetrate the hair shaft more effectively. Heat it very slightly in a non-metallic bowl over a pan of water. It should be no more than comfortably warm. Alternatively, wring out a towel in hot water and wrap it around your head – again ensuring that the heat is not uncomfortable – when you have applied the oil and again after massaging it in.

If you use a sauna or steam room, oil your hair before you go in and wrap it in a towel. This not only gives the oil a chance to penetrate more deeply, but it also protects the hair from the long-term drying effects of steam and heat.

hair and head massage

Why not combine an oil treatment for the scalp with a head massage, which Ayurveda recommends as part of your regular self-care routine? The series of movements aims to stimulate the body's systems, including glands, nerves and circulation, with anti-aging effects.

▽ **Gentle treatment brings out the best in fine flyway hair, so nurture it with the softest oil massage to help bring it back into balance.**

hair strengthening

If your hair is thinning or breaks easily, massage it with a strengthening herb-infused oil. This treatment is particularly recommended during pregnancy, to avoid the hair loss that plagues many women after childbirth.

ingredients

- 120 ml/4 fl oz/$\frac{1}{2}$ cup castor oil
- 550 ml/18 fl oz/$2\frac{1}{2}$ cups sesame or coconut oil
- 120 ml/4 fl oz/$\frac{1}{2}$ cup brahmi
- 120 ml/4 fl oz/$\frac{1}{2}$ cup amla
- 750 ml–1 litre/$1\frac{1}{4}$–$1\frac{3}{4}$ pints/3–4 cups water

Mix the castor oil with the sesame oil (for vata-type hair) or coconut oil (for pitta) and add the brahmi and amla. Stir with a wooden spoon until the herbs have blended into the oil (you can warm the oil a little to expedite the process). Leave overnight, then pour the herb-infused oil, with the water, into an enamelled or non-metallic pan. Bring to the boil and simmer until all the water has evaporated. Remove from the heat and allow to cool, then strain through muslin or cheesecloth.

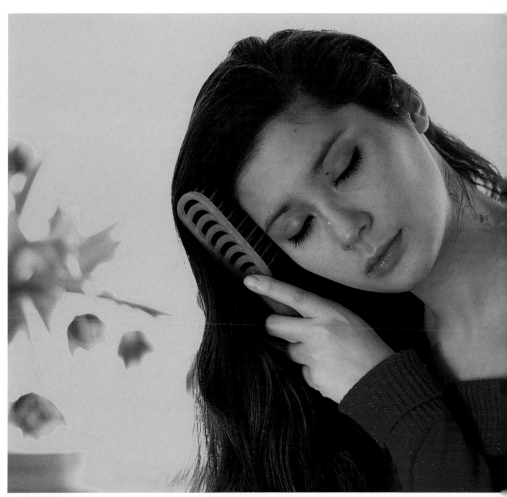

The art of henna

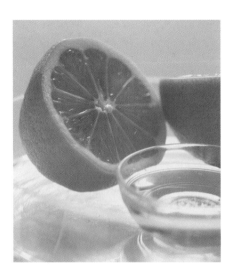

Henna is the classic Indian colourant for hair and skin. Before henna was cultivated in India, women stained their hands and feet with fruit dyes, but the arrival of henna from the Middle East, some time after AD 1000, allowed much greater artistry. Before a traditional wedding the bride's hands and feet are painted in intricate patterns, using a technique known as *mehendi*.

The dried stems and leaves are ground into a powder, then mixed with oil to form a paste, which is painted on the hands and feet with a slender stick and left for several hours, periodically moistened, during a special party for female friends and relatives. Dabbing with lemon juice and clove oil makes the colour darker and longer-lasting – an important point for the bride, since she is exempted from household chores until

THE RIGHT STUFF

Kits are available for an easy introduction to either hair dyeing or henna tattooing, but be wary of anything called "black henna". Some products contain chemicals such as PPD (p-Phenylenediamine) and silver nitrate, or even heavy metals. They give a darker, longer-lasting tattoo, but can cause violent skin reactions that may take days to appear – making a routine skin test useless.

◁ **Lemon brings out the bright colour of henna. For use on skin, strain the juice so that the paste will flow smoothly through the applicator.**

her wedding henna has worn off. After five hours or more the paste is allowed to dry, then scraped off. Today this is being taken up in Western countries as a form of body art.

following tradition

Today you can buy henna powder, and ready-mixed pastes are also available, though the results are not long-lasting and some may contain chemical additives. Henna is available with added dyes, but the natural orangey red gives the most striking colour on skin. For the best results draw a design on paper and follow this, as the paste makes a faint mark within moments and is hard to erase.

The design should stay visible for one to three weeks. To help it last longer, exfoliate the day before, and scrub the skin before you start. Afterwards, keep it moisturized with oil or hand cream. Pat dry after bathing and moisturize again. The colour will fade faster

if exposed to salt, chlorine and other chemicals (including harsh soaps), or if soaked in water.

hair conditioning

Henna is traditionally used to nourish the hair as well as revitalizing its colour. It has a cooling effect that helps to reduce excess pitta – which is seen as the cause of most hair and scalp problems. Henna can have a drying effect, so if you have dry hair it is best blended with oils or egg.

Indian women also add dried herbs – amla, aritha, brahmi, shikakai and triphala – for extra sheen. These are boiled in water, which is then strained and added to the henna paste.

Applying henna can be messy, and to get around this, Indian women apply the paste to sections of hair and wrap each section around the head before starting the next. The end result looks like a cocoon, and should stay in place.

▽ **Natural henna lends hair a vibrant auburn tint. Other herbs can be added to improve condition.**

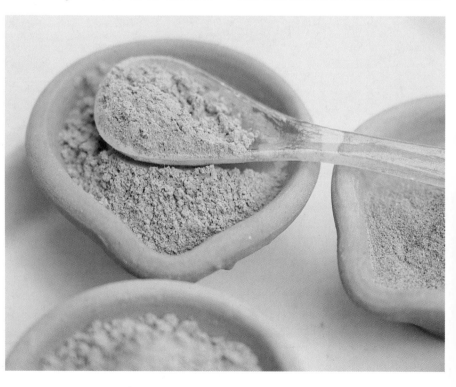

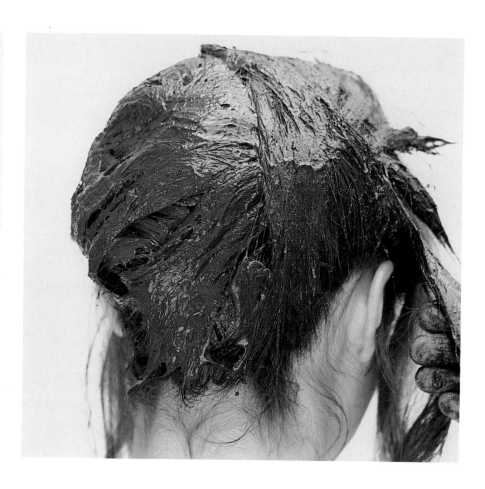

henna for hair

1 Mix natural henna powder to a paste with a little strong black tea, aiming for a consistency that will not slip off the hair. To soothe a dry scalp, add a beaten egg and/or yogurt. Leave the paste to stand for at least 3 hours.

▷ **2** Apply to the hair in sections, wrapping each around the head as you go. Dry the outside with a hairdryer and leave on for at least 2 hours, checking constantly that the paste has not dripped on to the skin, before washing it off thoroughly. (Note: it's best to wear gloves, to avoid staining your hands.)

henna for hands

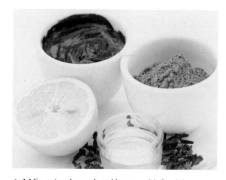

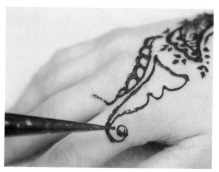

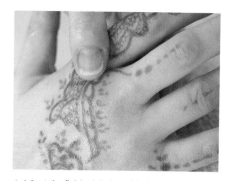

△ **1** Mix natural powdered henna with fresh lemon juice to make a thick paste. For a darker colour, add a little powdered cloves or a few drops clove oil (test on your inner arm first). Leave the paste for at least 3 hours, or overnight in cold weather. Also prepare a thick syrup of lemon juice and sugar and have ready a bowl each of lemon juice and clove oil (if suitable), with cotton balls.

2 Trace around your hand on paper and work out a design. When you're satisfied, copy it on to your hand using a non-toxic felt-tip pen.

△ **3** Add more lemon juice if necessary to make the paste just workable, then fill an applicator with a very fine nozzle. Apply, following the design you've drawn. Keep moistening the lines as you go along with dabs of lemon juice, followed by clove oil.

△ **4** Coat the finished design with the lemon syrup and cover with tissue paper, then with plastic wrap. Leave on for at least 6 hours, or overnight. Check it's dry, so that it won't smudge as you remove it, then pick off the paste. Moisturize with oil or hand cream.

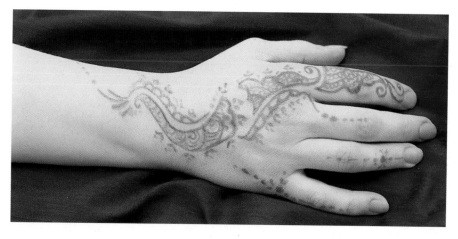

▷ **A skilled mehendi artist can create intricate designs full of symbolism. At home, start with a simple pattern that won't get smudged easily.**

Jewels – dare to dazzle

Adornment is part of everyday life in India, and it's full of meaning. Jewellery has always been popular: people didn't hide their wealth in banks but displayed it magnificently on every part of their body. For women, there was an economic benefit. In some eras a woman might be legally barred from owning anything except her clothes and jewellery – but these could be worth a rajah's ransom. Even the poorest women wore bangles as part of their everyday dress, and their cheerful jangling sound was said to represent laughter.

Gold was the favourite metal, as it was believed to purify everything it touched. Toe rings were made of silver or base metals, as it would have been disrespectful to put gold on the feet. Gold's nourishing qualities made it popular for those with vata dosha, whereas cool silver was considered more beneficial for pitta. Kapha was warmed by gold and copper.

Beads were traditionally used for their protective value as well as their prettiness. They were worn as talismans to protect against supernatural forces. Children wore "eye beads" to warn of the evil eye: if the child came under attack, it was believed, the beads would change colour or the thread would break as a warning.

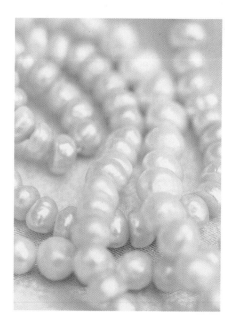

healing gems

In keeping with the all-encompassing philosophy of Ayurveda, jewels and gems were linked with human health and well-being in several ways. According to Indian astrology, they represented different planets and could modify the effects these had on people's lives.

In one expensive form of therapy, gems could be used to counteract diseases directly: reduced to ashes, they were blended into medicines known as *bhasmas*.

◁ **Pearls love to be worn regularly – their moon-soft glow dims if they're locked away. In return, they provide a cooling touch on hot pitta skin, or on any skin in hot weather.**

Diamonds, a powerful tonic for the heart, were also popular as an aphrodisiac. These days, people hoping to harness the virtues of jewels tend to use less drastic methods, instead leaving them in water overnight, so that the gem's energy is absorbed by the water, which they then drink.

Precious stones were also believed to have a balancing effect on the doshas. Blue sapphires, for example, could bring a dizzy vata mind back to earth, especially if set in gold. Cool pearls and diamonds set in silver reduced the heat of pitta. Kapha people were energized by clear crystals. Rubies, representing the sun, were so powerful that they could balance all three doshas, as well as promoting long life and vitality.

Ayurvedic practitioners recommend wearing an appropriate jewel in a setting that allows it to touch the skin. Today, Western doctors are well aware of the psychological benefits of therapies that lift the spirits, and who wouldn't feel better wearing a pair of diamond ear studs or a sapphire ring?

▽ **The beauty of anklets is enhanced by the delicate sound they make with each movement.**

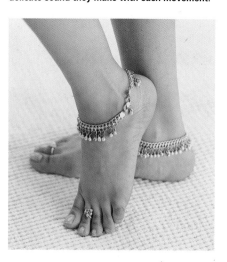

GEMS TO BALANCE YOUR DOSHA

Vata:	Pitta:	Kapha:
amethyst	pearl	amethyst
ruby	ruby	ruby
sapphire, blue or yellow	amethyst	clear quartz
lapis lazuli	blue sapphire	agate
red coral	red coral	beryl
topaz	beryl	white diamond
emerald	white diamond	lapis lazuli
jade	emerald	garnet
peridot	moonstone	cat's eye
citrine	clear quartz	blue sapphire
garnet	jade	opal
opal	peridot	jade

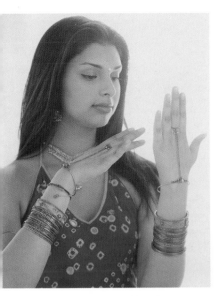

△ Layers of meaning: rings and bangles are a reminder of eternity, as well as adornment.

wedding ceremony. She also wears a *bindi*, or dot of vermilion pigment in the middle of her forehead, and regularly renews it for as long as her husband lives, to bring divine protection to the couple. Bindis are now worn by both married and single women, regardless of religious views. Instead of painting them on, women buy little fabric dots, decorated with glass or patterns.

Children may wear what at first glance looks like a bindi on their foreheads too, but for an entirely different reason. These are smudges of black, intended to deflect the attentions of evil spirits by marring the child's beauty.

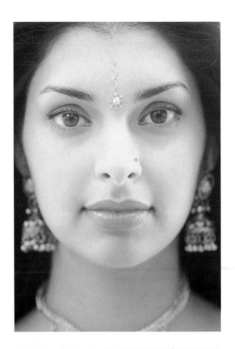

▷ The bindi, once just a dab of vermilion, has blossomed into an array of shapes and patterns.

bridal display

Traditional adornment sometimes shows a woman's marital status. Hair is worn with a central parting, which a married woman may decorate with a chain ending in a pendant on her forehead. Bangles are also signs of the married state in some parts of India, their never-ending circular shape representing eternity.

Never does a woman adorn herself more splendidly than at her wedding. A traditional bride wears 16 different kinds of jewellery: around her neck, in her hair, on her forehead, circling her waist and up her arms. They include earrings so heavy that they are supported by a chain over the ear as well as a hook through the lobe. She might wear a nose ring in the form of flowers, or a thumb ring set with a mirror. Finger or toe rings are connected to bracelets or anklets by a set of chains in the form of a lotus. Clusters of bells around her ankles ensure that her every movement wins attention.

protective colouring

Vermilion is the colour of the goddess Parvati, who protects married women and their husbands. In her honour, a married woman paints her hair parting with a vermilion powder called *sindoor*, which is first applied by the bridegroom during the

▷ Gold is the symbol of Lakshmi, goddess of wealth, and is held to purify everything it touches. Vata and kapha respond to its warmth.

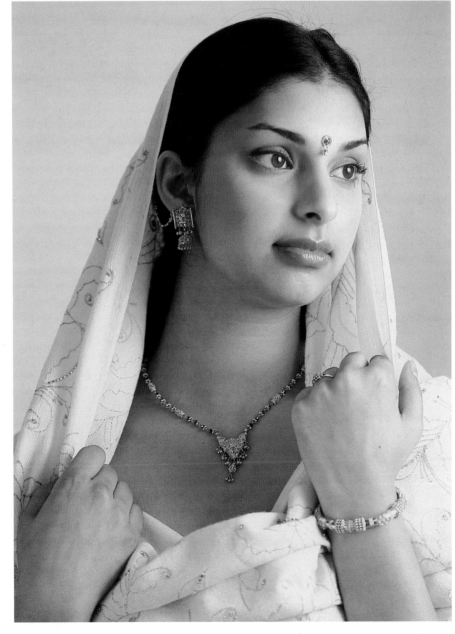

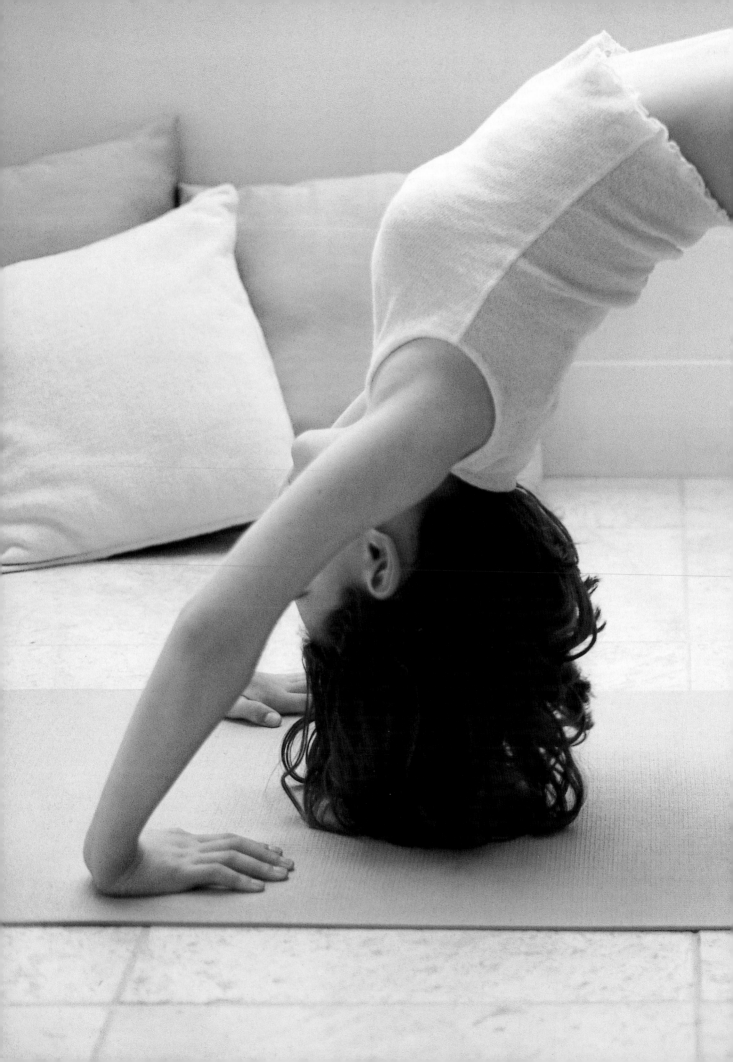

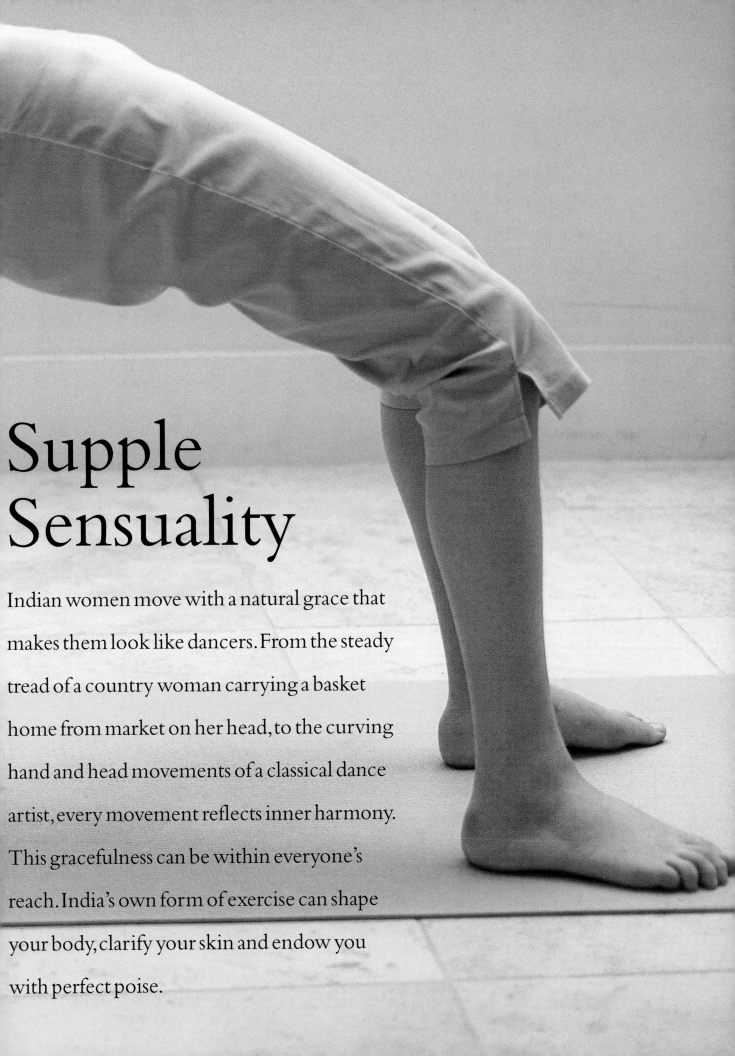

Supple Sensuality

Indian women move with a natural grace that makes them look like dancers. From the steady tread of a country woman carrying a basket home from market on her head, to the curving hand and head movements of a classical dance artist, every movement reflects inner harmony. This gracefulness can be within everyone's reach. India's own form of exercise can shape your body, clarify your skin and endow you with perfect poise.

Natural grace through yoga

As young children we all moved with unselfconscious grace, but from hunching over a school desk to slumping in front of a computer or television, many of us spend much of our lives with rounded shoulders and crumpled spines, and the heavy bags we carry often twist us to one side, too.

Most forms of exercise will help us look and feel better, but poor posture can sabotage a fitness regime, making exercise harder and leaving well-toned muscles further out of alignment than before. There is no such danger with yoga, and it is excellent for strengthening muscles and improving flexibility. In addition, its emphasis on lengthening and straightening the spine makes for perfect posture, creating an appearance of height and slenderness. Its regulated pattern of breathing lowers stress levels and eases tension from our faces as well as our bodies.

Yoga has become so popular in the West during the past few decades that we don't always remember where it came from. We

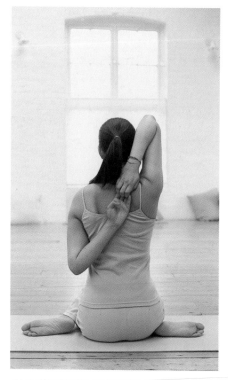

△ **Lengthening the spine and opening the chest is necessary if we are to help our cramped bodies regain a feeling of life.**

usually regard it as a set of flexibility exercises, or add it to a standard fitness regime as a stretch component. True, it is one of the best ways to build suppleness and delay the onset of old age. But yoga is far more than that, and in India it has always been closely linked with Ayurvedic medicine. Its name is Sanskrit for "union" or "connection": linking body, mind and the other non-physical levels to the universal mind. It has several elements, but the exercises generally practised in the West are what's called *hatha*, or physical, yoga.

Awareness of breathing is a central part of hatha yoga, and breath is synchronized with movement. Despite the effort you're putting in, this leads to a very calming, almost meditative rhythm that helps you push on through difficult parts. Pranayama – breathing exercises – form part of a standard yoga practice.

▽ **Working with a partner can help you keep your balance and move more confidently.**

SAFE MOVES

Hatha yoga was originally practised as an aid to meditation through controlling the body. Some movements, such as headstands, straight-legged body bends and backwards head rolls, can be dangerous for beginners. Others, such as stretches and twists, should not be forced. It's safest to learn from a qualified yoga teacher who has trained with one of the major organizations.

If you have health problems, don't take up any form of exercise before checking both with your own doctor and with an exercise expert who knows about medical contraindications. Yoga can bring great benefits to people with heart disease, back problems or arthritis, but they should take it up under the guidance of an instructor trained to work with these conditions.

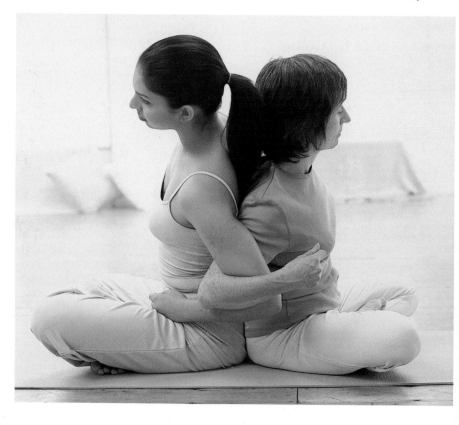

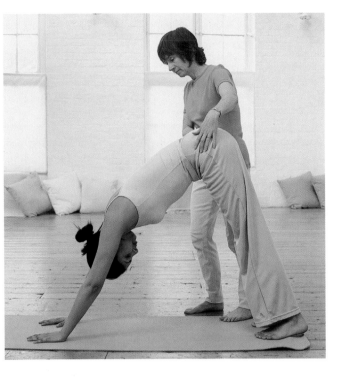

◁ **A good teacher will ask about any injuries or health problems, ensure you are holding the poses correctly and also help you come out of them safely.**

styles of hatha yoga

Yoga's dynamic strength allows it to adapt while retaining its essential meaning. In recent years it has changed from a faintly exotic pastime to an everyday event. It is offered in many new forms, some of which are rediscoveries of ancient techniques.

Ashtanga is a vigorous form that builds up intense heat, intended to purify the muscles and organs, expel impurities and release hormones to nourish the skin. The fast sequences originally kept warriors fit, and they're an all-round exercise for flexibility, strength and cardiovascular fitness. It is aimed at people who are already very fit.

Bikram yoga quickly attracted dancers and celebrities to its creator's Beverly Hills studio. The idea is that practising a stripped-down core of movements in a room heated to above body temperature allows the muscles to stretch more, while impurities are washed out on a tide of perspiration.

Contact yoga is practised with a partner, requiring good co-operation and balance. Advanced practitioners may be able to do a headstand on their partner's head, but most stick to supporting each other's back bends or aiding a little more stretch.

Dru yoga is a very gentle, peaceful form that includes relaxation and working as a group.

Iyengar yoga is the best known form outside India. Detailed poses, or *asanas*, are

▽ **Your teacher can help you to increase your stretch while staying within safe limits.**

carried out with great attention to technique. It can feel strenuous, but it is done in a slow, controlled manner that should allow you to stop if you feel you're pushing your muscles too far.

Jivamukti is fast-paced and rigorous, but also includes chanting and meditation to help maintain the balance between physical and spiritual.

Kundalini yoga is an esoteric form that aims for enlightenment through the release of energy up the spine. This is achieved through stretching, breathing exercises, chanting and meditation.

Sivananda yoga, one of the least strenuous forms, considers the physical exercises to be part of a holistic lifestyle. It includes meditation and promotes a feeling of peace.

Vini yoga emphasizes safe movements and individual tuition, letting you adapt poses to meet your ability rather than trying to force yourself into them.

Yoga Vanda Scaravelli is a gentle adaptation of Iyengar, focusing on the spine. It uses gravity and the breath to undo tension in the body and awaken the spine.

▽ **Keep the neck long as you look up, visualizing space between the vertebrae. Letting your head slump back could harm your spine.**

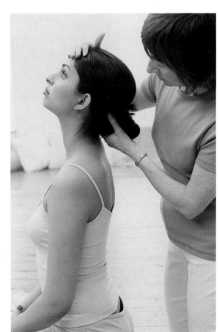

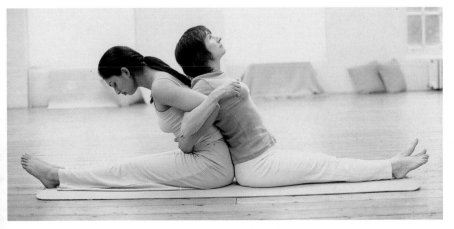

Find your fitness style

You don't need to read again that exercise is a vital component in any beauty regime. You may even be flipping guiltily past these pages, because you've come to see yourself as a hopeless fitness dropout. The Pilates class your friends rave about leaves you cold, and the last time you lifted a weight you felt like dropping it on the floor and running out of the gym. But don't despair: you could simply be following the wrong path for your dosha.

We all need to improve our cardiovascular fitness, increase flexibility, and build strength through weight-bearing exercise. But finding the right balance, and the right form of exercise, could be as simple as finding your true style. Even if you're perfectly content with your fitness routine – or lack of it – it's still worth considering whether you could make changes. When our energies are out of balance, we tend to slip further into the things that are causing the imbalance.

achieving balance

An energetic vata person may love running – an excellent and invigorating form of exercise. But when vata energy starts racing out of control, it's time to take another direction. Instead of arousing it further, turn to something slower and steadier, that will bring you safely back to earth.

A competitive pitta sportswoman may be way ahead of the field, but strangely unsatisfied by her achievement. Working up a daily sweat is just pouring fuel on her fiery nature. And it can be hard to persuade a relaxed kapha that exercise is a good thing when she feels fine without it.

It would be crazy to give up a form of exercise that you enjoy – it's hard enough for most of us to stick to a fitness programme. But Ayurveda suggests bringing more balance into your life, especially when your usual behaviour and routines are exacerbating any imbalances.

Sometimes our bodies instinctively know what's right for us at that moment, but sometimes we become set in ways that aren't the best. As you learn to know yourself better, you start to recognize the difference.

vata

You probably love lively exercise like dancing and running, but a typically speedy vata lifestyle can leave you feeling ungrounded. You also need to protect your joints from injury and build strength. As the most active of people, you're the least likely to need to join an aerobics class.

Bring your energies into balance with a steady, strengthening yoga style such as Vini. Iyengar is another good choice, so long as you're careful to recognize your current limits and don't risk harming vulnerable joints by excessive twisting or staying too long in a difficult weight-bearing pose. Instead of trying to force a stretch, let your muscles relax as you sink into a feeling of unhurried calm.

Walking, t'ai chi and Pilates are other useful exercises for you. Add some form of weight-training: the repetitive movements will leave your ever-active mind free to work out a new theory while you tone your abdominals. If these options sound slow and boring, give them a chance. As you become accustomed to this challenge you should start noticing a new smoothness in your movement as well as in your muscles.

▽ **Muscle-toning exercises such as Pilates are useful for vatas, whose high-speed metabolism makes aerobic exercise less of a necessity.**

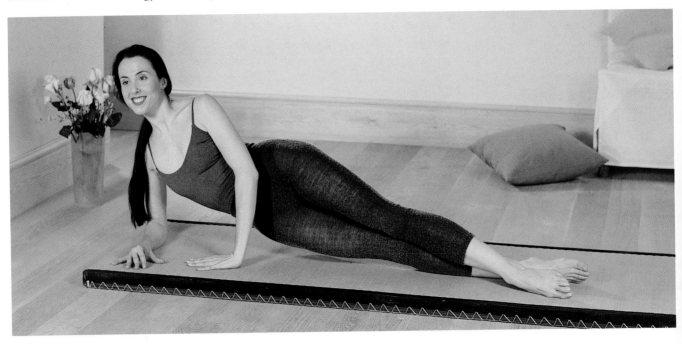

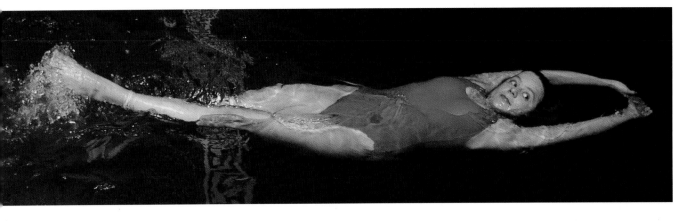

pitta

Your competitive instincts lead you towards races and sports, but you need to avoid overheating, whether from exertion, a hot room or the midday sun. You could benefit from all yoga styles that increase flexibility without making you sweat. Concentrate on lengthening your muscles or easing gently into a deeper stretch without force or jerky movements, as in the yoga of Vanda Scaravelli. Working with a partner could help develop your co-operative instincts. The gentle routines of Dru or Sivananda yoga will promote feelings of peace that you may not have known for some time.

Swimming is ideal for your hot-blooded nature: the water helps balance your energies while you focus on your own steady progress. Cold-climate holidays give you a chance to enjoy skiing or snowboarding. Day to day, you need a moderate amount of exercise, with long walks providing an easy option.

kapha

You're naturally strong and healthy, and don't particularly like exercise, but you still need to build up flexibility and cardiovascular fitness. Though you reap the psychological benefits of taking life at a calm, steady pace, you need to build some energetic exercise into your routine.

With yoga, you're most likely to be motivated by a high-speed form that's fun and gets your body pumping out endorphins. Try Ashtanga or Jivamukti, which will also counteract your tendency to gain weight.

Any high-energy exercise class will give you the lively workout you need. Your strength makes you an asset in team sports, or you could take a salsa course.

△ **Swimming is the perfect exercise for pittas: it's a rhythmic, calming motion that lets them work off plenty of energy without overheating.**

▽ **Anyone with kapha tendencies can have fun getting their exercise, and their stamina keeps them on the dance floor when others flag.**

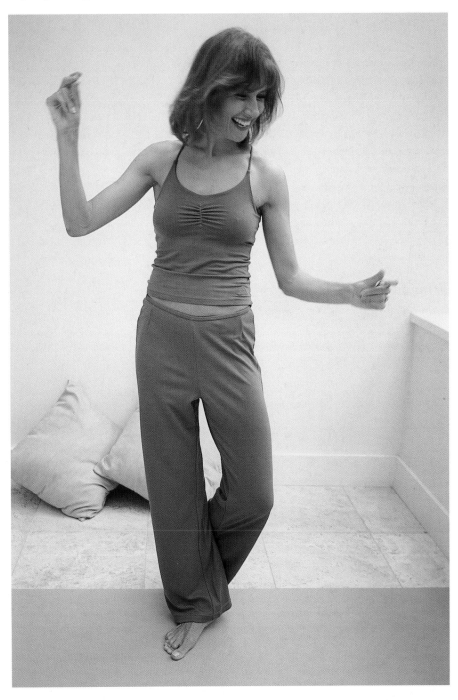

Move like a dancer

For most of us, brief bouts of exercise are interspersed with long hours of sedentary work, slumped in a chair and barely turning our heads. The effects show in our skin, our tired eyes and even our speech, from throats too constricted to allow our voices to be full and resonant.

All forms of yoga increase suppleness, allowing us to move more freely with a natural sensuality. Once we start practising yoga, the effects spread far beyond the hour spent twisting and stretching in the class. Straightening and lengthening the spine becomes a beneficial habit, changing the way we sit, stand, walk and talk. We hold our head level, as if suspended from the ceiling by a string, and the chin neither sags nor juts.

The asanas described on these pages are suitable for all doshas and are especially valuable for improving posture. In all cases you're aiming to lengthen and straighten your spine and limbs to rediscover a naturally upright stance.

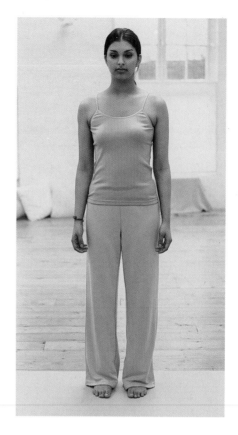

the Mountain (Tadasana)

◁ **1** Stand with feet parallel and a little apart, arms by your sides. Lift and spread your toes, then plant them firmly on the floor. Keep your legs strong by feeling the front thigh muscles pulling up towards your groin. Tuck in your tailbone so that the front of your pelvis feels slightly higher than the back.

2 Lengthen your spine upwards while letting your shoulders and arms relax backwards and down. Imagine your head supported by a string from the centre of your scalp; your chin is level, leaving your throat comfortably open without compressing the back of your neck. Let your face relax.

3 Open your chest, without forcing your shoulders rigidly back. Let your stomach gently swell as breath fills your lungs, then tighten the abdominal muscles and expel all the stale air.

Standing Side Stretch (Ardha Chandrasana)

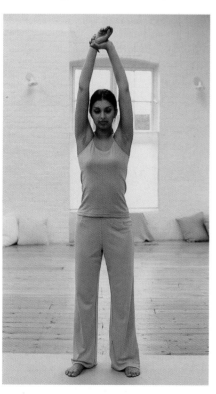

◁ **1** Starting in Mountain pose, take your feet a little further apart and slowly raise your arms above your head as you breathe in. Grasp your right wrist with your left hand as you breathe out.

▷ **2** On the next inbreath, lean to the left, facing forwards and bending sideways from the waist. Don't let your head, arms or torso flop; hold the position strongly and feel strength radiating from your fingers. Return to the centre on an outbreath and repeat on the other side, holding your left wrist.

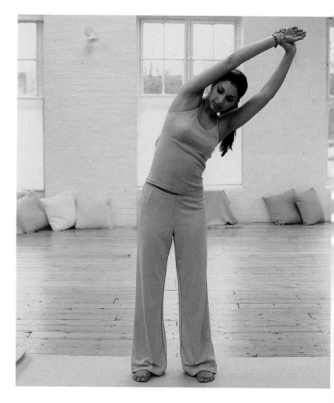

the Tree (Vrksasana)

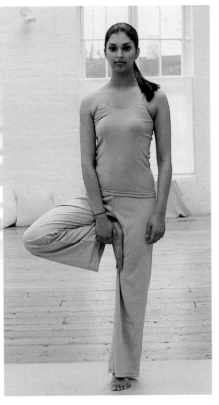 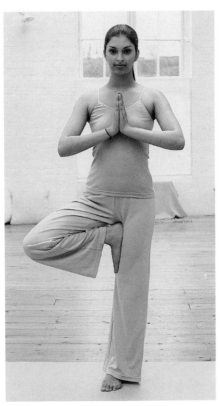 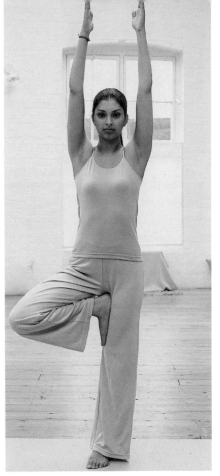

△ **1** Standing straight and looking straight ahead, take a moment to feel balanced and firmly rooted. Bending your right leg, place your foot as close to the top of your inside left thigh as you can comfortably reach, lifting it into position with your right hand if you wish. Stretch your right knee out to the side.

△ **2** To help keep your balance, fix your gaze on something motionless at about eye level. Spread out the toes of your left foot to grip the floor firmly. Breathing in, put your palms together with fingers pointing upwards as if making the Indian greeting *Namaste*. Try to hold this position for about 5 seconds, breathing naturally.

△ **3** On an inbreath stretch your arms straight above your head and turn your palms inwards. Feel the stretch from your raised hands to your feet, and the energy travelling the length of your body. Aim to hold for up to 20 seconds, breathing naturally. On an outbreath, bring your hands down, first to Namaste level, then down by your sides. Return your right foot to the floor and stand for a moment feeling grounded. Then repeat the exercise on the other side.

the Cow (Gomukhasana)

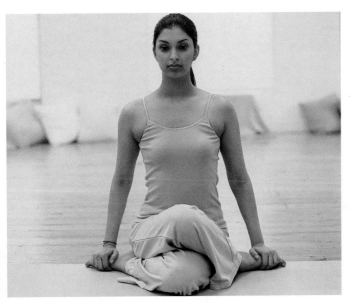 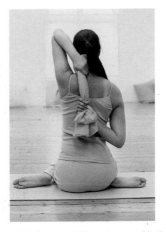

△ **1** Tuck your left heel beside your right buttock, trying to keep the knee on the floor. Cross the right knee over that leg and bring the right foot round beside you. If you find this difficult, sit with legs crossed and concentrate on the arm movements.

△ **2** Relax your right arm by your side then, on an inbreath, bring the right hand up between your shoulderblades. On the next inbreath, raise the left arm as if reaching for the ceiling. On the outbreath, bring your left hand down and try to grasp the right hand. If (like most of us) you can't reach at first, hold each end of a scarf. Hold the posture for around 10 seconds, breathing naturally, then on an inbreath raise the left hand again and bring both hands down beside you as you breathe out. Uncross your legs and stretch them out. Repeat on the other side.

Beauty from within

Why does your skin glow so beautifully when you surface from a swimming pool or return from a brisk walk? Any exercise that stimulates the circulation brings fresh oxygenated blood to the face, instantly enlivening the complexion. The long-term effects of regular exercise are just as clear – keeping the complexion fresh and strengthening the muscles that support the skin. The high-energy forms of yoga give your complexion a healthy boost that lasts long after you've showered and cooled down, but yoga's range of asanas includ[es] several that stimulate circulation to the he[ad] without working up a sweat. Hold each [of] the poses for around 30 seconds, or as long [as] feels comfortable, and come out of them [by] retracing the steps described.

Downward-facing Dog (Adho Mukha Shvanasana)

In this position you should feel a stretch in your back and the backs of your legs, but don't force it, and don't try it without an instructor if you have trouble with your knees or lower back. If you're not very fit you may feel dizzy when you put your head down, so adapt the pose until you feel comfortable. (If the dizziness persists whenever you try this kind of exercise, get your doctor to check your heart and blood pressure.)

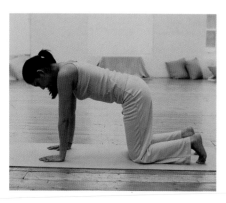

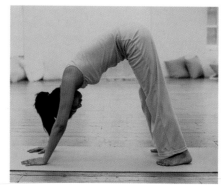

◁ **2** As you breathe out, try to straighten your legs by lifting your hips up and back. Keep your shoulde[rs] relaxed and breathe naturally. Your head should remain in line with your spine, not flopping down or pushed back. If you can straighten your legs withou[t] forcing your knees uncomfortably, increase the stretch by lowering your heels towards the floor. O[n] an outbreath, try to lengthen your spine by bringing your hips further up and back.

△ **1** Kneel on all fours, with hips directly above knees and shoulders above wrists. Take time to feel well grounded, with toes tucked in below heels and fingers spread out, firmly gripping the floor.

the Lion (Simhasana)

This is a wonderful way of exercising your face, improving both circulation and muscle support. It firms the muscles of the face and neck, keeping wrinkles at bay.

▷ Sit with your legs crossed or kneel in a comfortable upright position. Rest your hands on your knees. As you breathe out spread your fingers wide apart, open your eyes as wide as you can and look up towards the centre of your forehead. Stick your tongue out and down as far as possible. Breathe out hard, making a loud, forceful "hah" sound. As you breathe in, draw in your tongue and relax your eyes and hands.

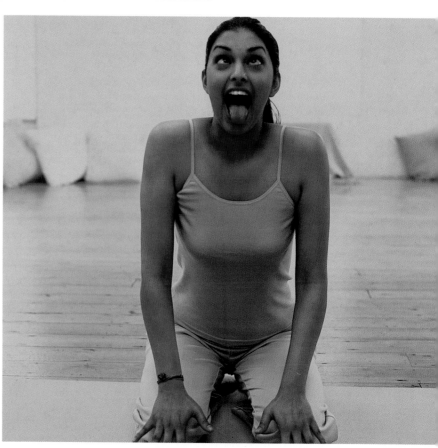

Standing Forward Bend (Uttanasana)

This useful asana revitalizes the complexion, tones the leg muscles, calms nerves and reduces vata energy.

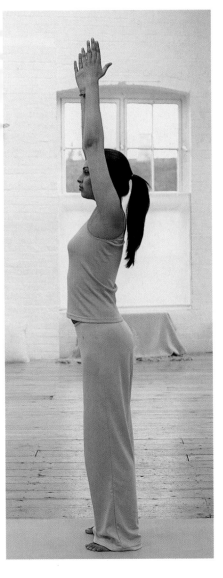

◁ **1** Stand in Mountain pose, then move your feet shoulder-width apart. Breathe in and raise both arms above your head with palms facing in, feeling the spine stretch upwards.

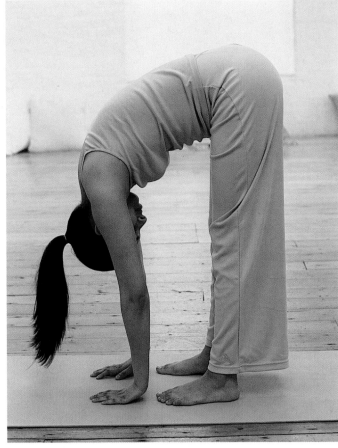

△ **2** Breathe out as you bring your torso and arms slowly forward in a straight line, hinging from the hips and (to keep your back flat) leading with the chest. Go down as far as you can without straining your back. Keep the movement controlled to avoid harming your back, and bend your knees if necessary. Stay down as long as you feel comfortable, up to 30 seconds, breathing naturally, then, on an inbreath, bend your knees and unroll your spine vertebra by vertebra to come slowly up.

the Child (Murha Janusasana)

As well as improving circulation to the face and head, this is a very relaxing pose that eases the spine, making it ideal to follow more strenuous asanas.

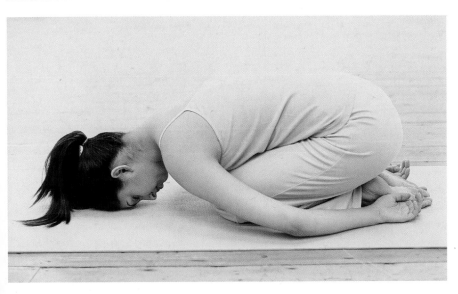

1 Kneel on the floor, sitting on your heels with legs together, arms relaxed by your sides and spine erect. As you breathe in, stretch your spine upwards as if pulled by a string from the top of your head and feel your chest and diaphragm expanding.

◁ **2** Breathing out, bring your body forwards face first, hinging from the hips without hunching the back. Bring your head down on to your knees or the floor in front. Rest your arms beside your body, palms up, on top of your feet if you can reach that far. Breathe naturally and feel your spine relax. This is a relaxation pose that you can hold for a couple of minutes, as long as you feel comfortable, before coming slowly up.

Body shaping

A sensuous shape relies on well-toned muscles. That means some kind of strength-building work, but many forms of strengthening exercise, such as weight-training, can create rather chunky muscles. Adding some stretch exercise is vital if you want to firm up without adding bulk, a fitness instructors always warn. The stretching element is built into yoga.

the Cat (Chakravakasana)

This tones muscles in the back, arms and buttocks and stretches the hamstrings.

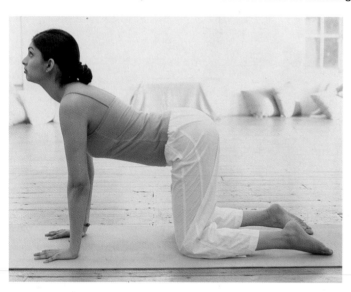

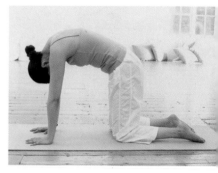

◁ **1** Kneel on all fours with shoulders above wrists, hips above knees and soles facing upwards. As you breathe in, arch your back downwards so that your waist sinks lower than your hips and shoulders. Lift your head, without tipping it back – the length of your neck should be maintained.

△ **2** As you breathe out, come back to a central position. Continuing the outbreath, arch your back upwards and tuck your chin in towards your chest. Breathe in as you return to the central position and on to arch your back downwards. Repeat this movement slowly several times.

the Cobra (Bhujangasana)

This tones buttock muscles and pectorals. Don't risk damaging your neck by tipping your head too far back in this or any other backwards bend.

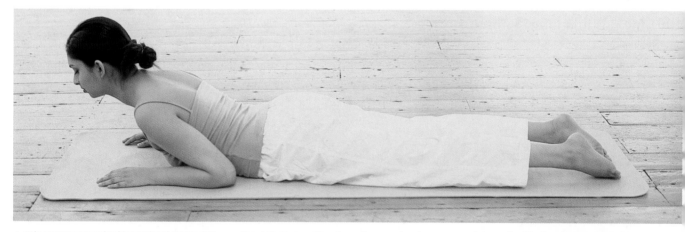

△ **1** Lie on your stomach with your head on one side resting on the floor, legs stretched out, with the soles of the feet pointing upwards, and arms by your side with palms upwards. Bend your arms and bring your hands beside your shoulders and, as you breathe in, slowly raise your chest. Keep your elbows beside your body, shoulders down and chest moving forwards. On an outbreath, push your palms down and raise your upper body as far as possible while keeping your pubic bone in contact with the floor. Look straight ahead, feeling the front of your body opening and expanding.

2 As you breathe in, raise your head slightly and direct your gaze upwards, but without tipping your head backwards. Relax the muscles in your back and buttocks, and feel your spine lengthen. Breathe naturally. Lower your gaze and look straight ahead again, then slowly lower your upper body to the starting position.

the Bridge (Setu Bandha)

In this asana, you're working on your hips and thighs.

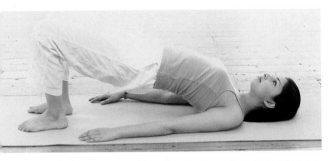

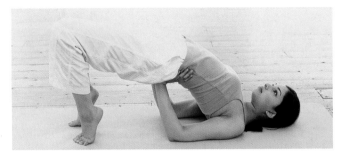

1 Lie on your back, arms by your sides with palms facing downwards. Bring your heels towards your torso, hip-width apart. As you breathe in, raise your buttocks as high as possible, pushing upwards with your pelvis till you are resting on your feet and shoulders. Tuck your chin in and let your head rest on the floor.

△ **2** If this is very easy, try an advanced version: with upper arms on the floor, bend your elbows and as you breathe out put your hands under your waist for support. Do not flop down on to your hands or push your spine up too high. If it's hard to keep your back raised, come down gently.

Lying-down Twist (Jathara Parivartanasana)

This works on trimming the waist while releasing tension from muscles in the back.

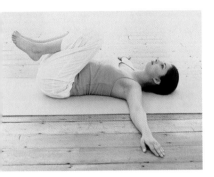

▷ **2** On an outbreath, lower your knees to the floor on one side and turn your head to the other. Hold for as long as is comfortable, then slowly come back to the centre on an outbreath, pause for a moment and repeat on the other side.

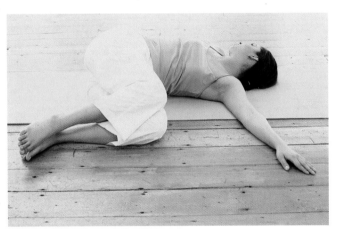

△ **1** Lie on the floor with arms outstretched, palms down. Bend your knees and raise them to your chest. Keep your neck and spine in a straight line.

the Warrior (Virabhadrasana) I, with arms raised

This pose tones the thighs, calves and chest.

1 Stand in Mountain pose, then move your feet sideways until they are about twice hip-width apart. Breathe in and turn your right foot through a quarter-circle to the right, placing your right heel in line with the left instep. Breathe out and rotate your body from the hips to face right.

▷ **2** Bend your right leg so that your knee forms a right angle, keeping the knee directly above the heel. Breathe in and raise your arms above your head until your hands are shoulder-width apart with palms facing in. Push your feet firmly into the floor and stretch up. Breathe out and lift your head slightly, without tipping it back, to look upwards. Breathe naturally and hold for a few seconds.

3 On an inbreath, lower your head again so that you are looking ahead. As you breathe out, bring your arms down by your sides, straighten your right leg and turn

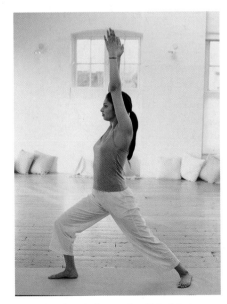

your body to face the front again, with both feet pointing forwards. Keeping your legs wide apart, repeat the movements on the other side.

the Warrior II, with arms outstretched

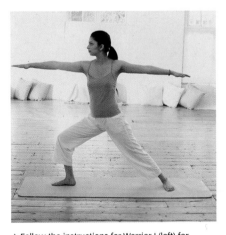

△ Follow the instructions for Warrior I (left) for the leg movements for this version, but do not turn your body to the right or raise your arms above your head. Instead, trying to keep hips facing squarely forwards, stretch both arms out with palms facing down. Turn your head only, to look along your outstretched right arm.

Dynamic vitality

Different asanas can help you relax or feel more energetic, improve concentration or calm your mind. Calming poses include those where the body closes in on itself, such as the Forward Bends and the Child. For a surge of energy, you should work through dynamic positions such as the Lightning Bolt and the Warrior. Balancing asanas such as the Tree and the Eagle aid concentration and the Warrior poses promote inner strength. Any of the poses that release tension, such as the Lying-down Twist or the Dog, can aid relaxation. But the classic relaxer is the Corpse.

The way you breathe is almost as important in yoga as the way you move. Keep your respiration steady and match your movements to the flow of breath, breathing in with an upward or outward movement, out as you go down or sink deeper into a stretch. You soon start to notice how it helps you keep a rhythm to your movements. Aim to breathe out slightly more than you breathe in.

Breathing exercises, or pranayama ("controlling the life force"), form part of a yoga routine. In the Ayurvedic view, the breath carries the prana, or life force, around the body in thousands of channels; pranayama helps keep this flow steady and unobstructed. Because one of the main channels runs down the spine, good posture helps keep it clear.

Seated Forward Bend (Paschimottanasana)

▷ Sit upright on your tailbone with your legs together and straight out in front of you, toes up. On an outbreath, fold forwards from the hips to hold your ankles or your toes, without hunching your back. Ideally, keep your legs straight and bring your head down towards your knees, but let your knees bend if your back hurts, and don't force yourself to reach further than is comfortable. Hold for up to 30 seconds, then slowly return, on an inbreath, to an upright sitting position.

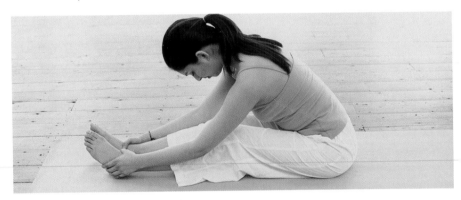

the Lightning Bolt (Utkatasana)

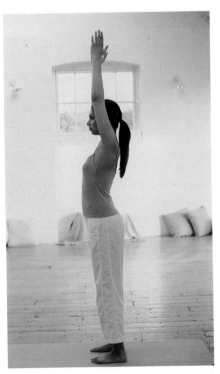

◁ **1** Start in Mountain pose, then breathe in as you raise your arms above your head. Breathe out and bend your knees. They should be no further forward than directly above your toes. Let your body slant naturally forwards, without rounding your back.

▷ **2** Be careful not to let your knees buckle inwards. Extend the arms in line with your torso. Breathe deeply three or four times, feeling the energy of the lightning bolt that your body forms from fingertips to toes. On an inbreath, return to Mountain pose.

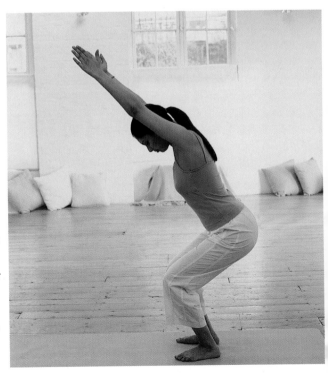

he Eagle (Garudasana)

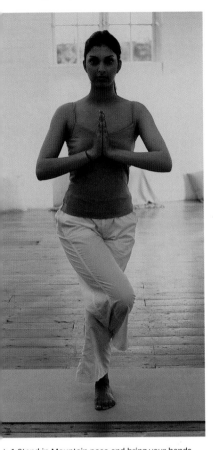

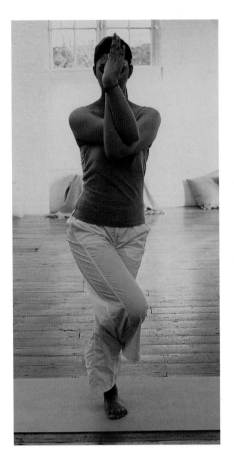

△ **1** Stand in Mountain pose and bring your hands into Namaste position. On an inbreath, bend your knees and wrap the right leg around the left, trying to hook your foot behind the ankle. To aid balance, focus your gaze on something still at eye level. Beginners can stay in Mountain pose and do the arm movements only.

△ **2** Keeping your shoulders relaxed, raise your arms in front of your shoulders on the next inbreath and cross the right elbow over the left. With thumbs at eye level, bring the palms together. Remain still, gazing at the thumbs and breathing normally. Be aware of the feeling of opening and stretching across your upper back; this is also excellent for relieving stiff shoulders.

the Corpse (Savasana)

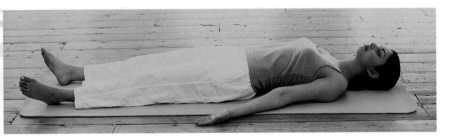

△ Just as it sounds: lie on your back, arms by your sides with palms upwards and legs outstretched. Relax and let your feet roll outwards as your head seems to sink into the floor. If this makes your lower back ache, bend your knees upwards.

A BALANCED PRACTICE
Remember to use counter-poses: if you do a strenuous asana such as the Eagle, follow it with something gentle like the Child. Any pose that involves a movement to the right or left should be carried out in pairs, so that both sides of the body get equal benefit and stay in balance.

OVERBREATHING
If you become dizzy you've been breathing in too deeply. Give a long outward breath, then breathe in and out of a paper bag a few times to re-establish the correct levels of oxygen and carbon dioxide.

cleansing breath (kapalabhati)

This cleanses the entire respiratory system and freshens the skin. It also strengthens the muscles of the abdomen and aids digestion. It is considered so cleansing that its Sanskrit name means "making your skull shine". If you practise it every day your face should shine with health.

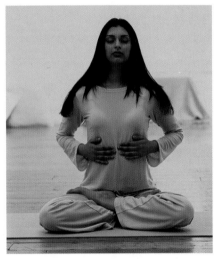

△ Sit with your back straight and breathe out hard in a series of short sharp exhalations through the nose. Tighten your stomach muscles as you breathe out, squeezing air out of your lungs. You won't need·to make any effort to breathe in: when you relax the stomach muscles air will flow into the lungs naturally. After the tenth inbreath, breathe out for as long as you can and try to empty the lungs. Take a few normal breaths before doing another set.

bee breath (brahmari)

This is a relaxing technique that can send even insomniacs to sleep. It can also give you a deliciously sexy voice, releasing tension in the throat that causes harshness or squeakiness.

Sit upright, close your eyes and let a long outbreath lead naturally to a long inhalation. Breathing through your nose, make a continuous humming sound each time you breathe out. Relax and let it become a deep, rich sound. Focus your mind on this sound, which should continue the whole time you're breathing out.

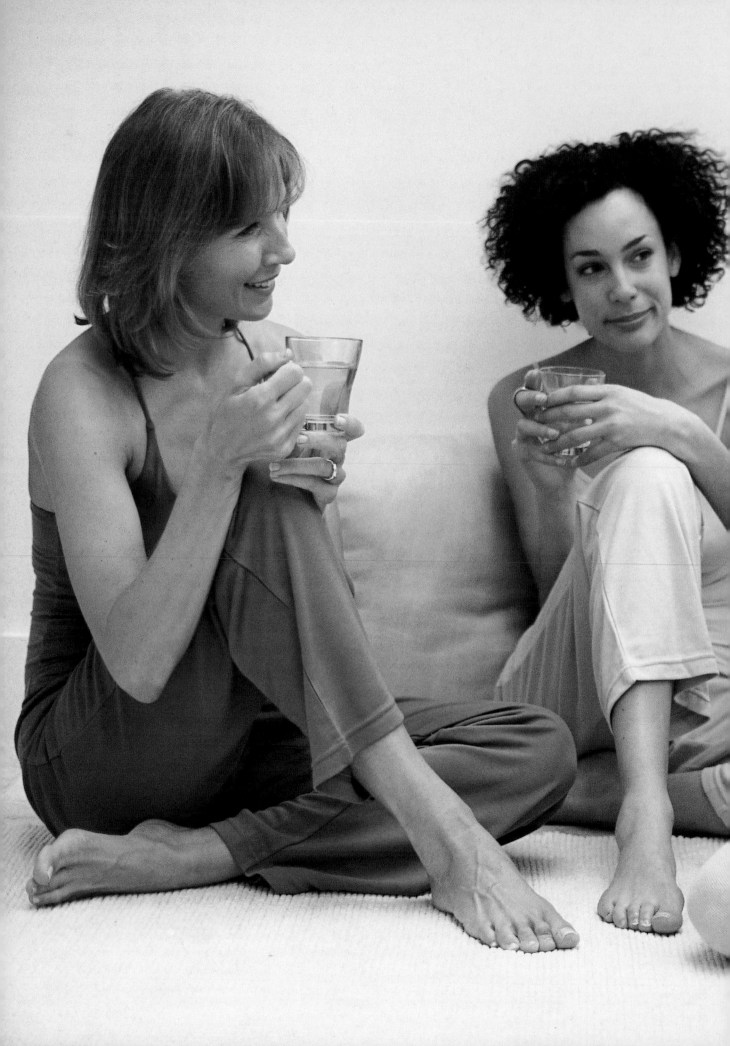

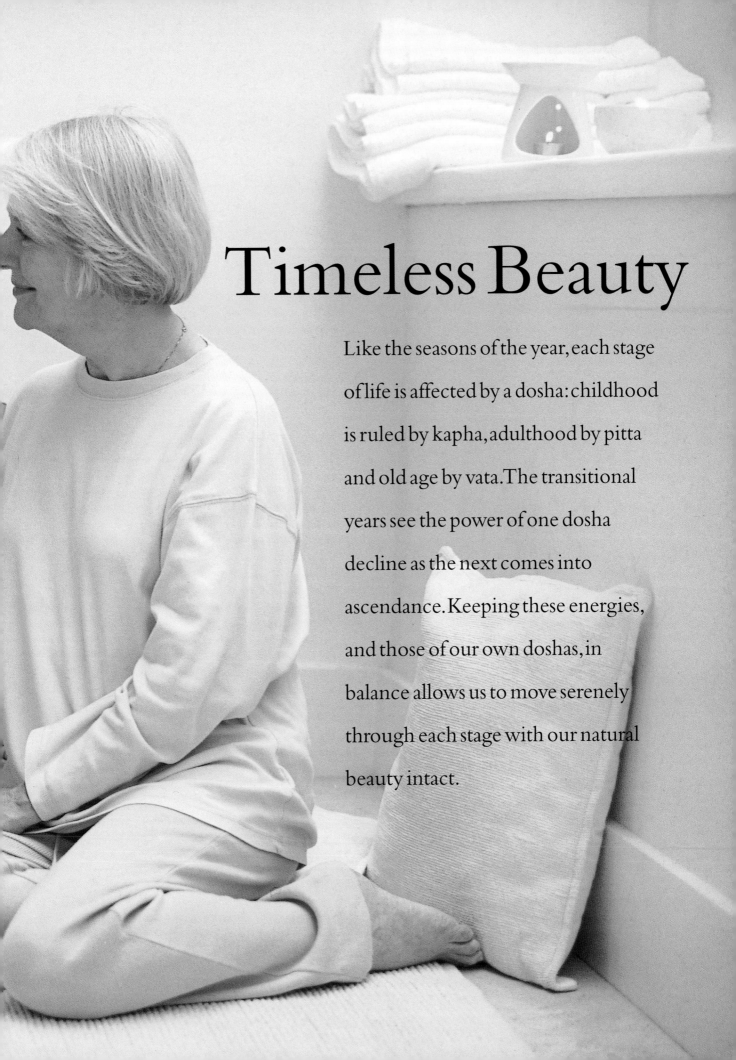

Timeless Beauty

Like the seasons of the year, each stage of life is affected by a dosha: childhood is ruled by kapha, adulthood by pitta and old age by vata. The transitional years see the power of one dosha decline as the next comes into ascendance. Keeping these energies, and those of our own doshas, in balance allows us to move serenely through each stage with our natural beauty intact.

The teenage transition

As children we had kapha's perfect skin, placid outlook and natural grace – not that we cared. Within a few years we're wondering what happened to those desirable attributes and wishing we could get them back. But by then we're already moving on into the pitta stage, which will last until the menopause.

Transitions are always a challenge, and – after birth – adolescence is the first big one. With depressive kapha and fiery pitta energies in conflict, our moods lurch from rage to despair. Since blood is a pitta element, the start of a period banishes premenstrual syndrome by reducing excessive pitta energy – but then hormonal changes make the skin erupt with acne and the hair turn lank. In Ayurvedic terms, the last burst of kapha energy turns skin into an oil well, ready to be ignited by pitta's fire. The body's toxic load of ama builds up too, and can find no way out except into the skin.

We slouch to disguise our embarrassing new height and breast shape (or lack of it) and loss of self-confidence can lead to problems such as eating disorders. Yet this is also a time of excitement and discoveries as we move towards independence. Ayurveda's holistic teachings show us how to be our best now, and at every stage of life. The earlier we start, the more radiant health and confidence we gain to carry us through challenging stages.

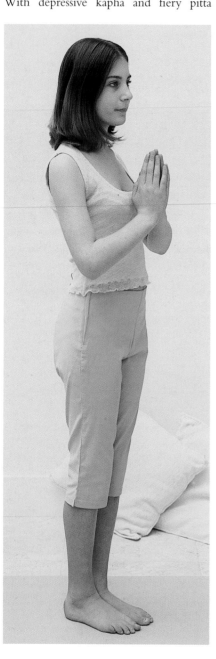

Yoga routine

Carrying out this set of asanas every day should help clear your skin, keep your weight steady and give your body image a healthy boost. When you have time and energy, do all the positions instead of making choices. Keep your movements strong, feeling the energy coursing through your body and out to the tips of your fingers and toes.

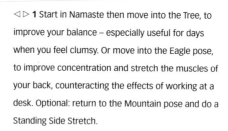

◁ ▷ **1** Start in Namaste then move into the Tree, to improve your balance – especially useful for days when you feel clumsy. Or move into the Eagle pose, to improve concentration and stretch the muscles of your back, counteracting the effects of working at a desk. Optional: return to the Mountain pose and do a Standing Side Stretch.

2 Try the Warrior pose, to shape legs and increase inner strength, helping you cope with mood swings and PMS, or the Lightning Bolt, for more energy.

3 Perform the Forward Bend, staying down for as long as you feel comfortable – up to 30 seconds – to stretch your hamstrings and bring fresh oxygenated blood to your face to clear skin blemishes.

4 Lie down and perform the Cobra.

5 Turn over and move into the Lying-down Twist, to tone your waist and let your hips swing as you walk.

6 Move into the Corpse. While you're relaxing after your workout, try to let your mind go blank and feel as if you're sinking into the floor.

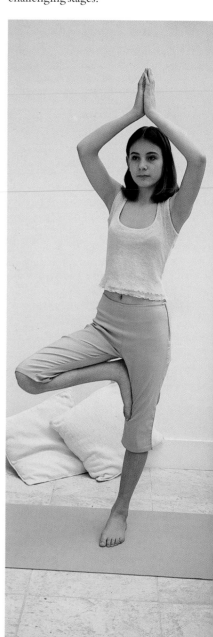

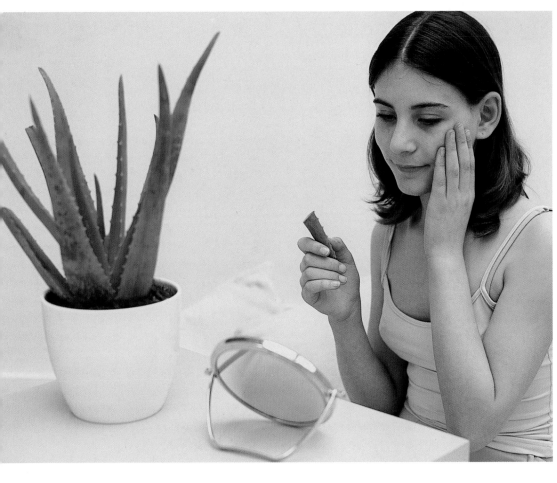

◁ Soothe spots and inflamed skin with the juicy pulp from an aloe vera leaf. It will leave your face feeling clean and supple.

eed your face

he skin blemishes that disfigure the eenage years are caused by an excess of apha and, especially, pitta energies. Kapha ncreases oiliness, leading to blackheads, while pitta energy causes inflammation and ruptions. These can be counteracted by voiding the rich, fried and highly spiced oods that aggravate pitta and – to a lesser xtent – the sweet or salty foods that do the same to kapha. To reduce ama, eat food as fresh and unprocessed as possible. Junk food breaks most of the laws of Ayurveda and has cruel effects on teenage skin.

teenage skincare

When skin erupts, it's natural to feel desperate and scrub it with chemicals, but these often make matters worse. Instead, just keep skin normally clean and resist the urge to touch it. Dab spots with cream made from the antiseptic leaves of the neem tree – then leave them alone. For a very simple remedy, keep an aloe vera plant to break tips off, or buy the pure pulp. Fresh air is good for your skin, but don't sunbathe. Strong sunlight slows down oil production temporarily, but it may then go into overdrive to compensate. Skin cancer is a greater risk if you've been sunburnt in your teens.

SKINCARE RECIPES

Each of these soothing preparations for troubled skin should be spread over the face and left for 15–30 minutes while you relax. Rinse off thoroughly with warm water and splash with a gentle toner such as rose water.

FOR OILY SKIN:

• Beat an egg white until it is fluffy and add 5 ml/1 tsp tangerine juice.

• Mix 2.5 ml/½ tsp honey with 10 ml/2 tsp lemon juice. Mix to a paste with multani mitti (fuller's earth) and a little rose water. This should be removed after 15 minutes.

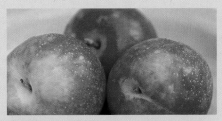

△ Combat acne with plums mashed in almond oil.

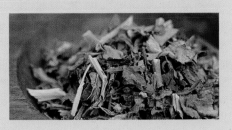

FOR ACNE:

• Boil 6 plums until soft, remove the skins and mash the pulp with 5 ml/1 tsp almond oil.

• Mix 5 ml/1 tsp each sandalwood powder and turmeric with enough milk to make a paste.

• Mix 5 ml/1 tsp either nutmeg or ground cumin seeds with water and spread on the affected areas only.

• Make a paste of fenugreek leaves and water, and spread on acne-prone areas. This can help prevent spots appearing.

◁ Fenugreek is used as a purifying herb – on the skin as well as in food.

Adult life: staying on top

Adulthood is pitta, ruled by the fiery dosha whose energetic influence sees us through our many tasks and responsibilities, not the least of which are the bearing and raising of children. At the busiest time of our lives, overwork can trigger a pitta imbalance, manifesting itself as irritability, impatience and heartburn.

dinacharya

Routines are a central part of Ayurveda, which teaches that living to a rhythm helps to keep us in tune with the energies inside and around us. Establishing an Ayurvedic routine, or *dinacharya*, is the first step to bringing the energies back into balance. It also makes it easier to sleep, exercise and eat healthily, helping to keep your weight steady and your skin clear.

• Wake up early – if not before sunrise, at least an hour before you have to leave home. Take a couple of minutes to visualize the day ahead and see it all going smoothly, then get up within about five minutes of waking.
• Give yourself a brief whole-body massage. If you use oil, leave it on for about 20 minutes before showering.
• Take 10–20 minutes to meditate and do some breathing exercises.
• Wash or shower, and splash your face and eyelids with cold water after cleansing.

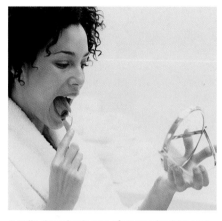

△ **Daily cleansing is part of staying healthy, and gently scraping the tongue freshens your mouth.**

Clean your tongue with a special scraper, or use the edge of a teaspoon (kept for that purpose only).
• Drink a glass of water, cool or warm but not ice-cold, to aid digestion and help keep skin fresh.
• Do your yoga routine now if possible.
• Don't leave home without eating any breakfast. Clean your teeth and tongue after you have eaten, and try to do the same after every meal.
• Drink water throughout the day so you

never feel thirsty. However, it's best not [to] drink while you're eating.
• Have a good meal – preferably your mai[n] meal – at lunchtime. Eat mindfully, takin[g] time to enjoy your food.
• Get some active exercise and some ment[al] stimulation each day. If you work at a des[k] go for a run or attend an exercise class. [If] you're running after children all day, read [a] book when you have a moment to yoursel[f].
• If you didn't have time to do yoga in th[e] morning, do it before dinner. Otherwis[e] meditate then.
• Eat a light evening meal, preferably early.
• Do 10–20 minutes' meditation if yo[u] didn't do this before eating.
• Go for a walk after you've eaten.
• Go to bed in time to allow yourself enoug[h] sleep. Most people need nine hours a nigh[t] in their teens, decreasing to eight in the[ir] 20s, about seven in the 40s and an hour [or] so less in old age.

You'll be impressive if you stick to th[is] routine every day – especially with childre[n] around. But using it as a basis helps you st[ay] in control of your time and energy.

▷ **Balance your mental and physical routine. Read a book if you're always on your feet; go for a run if you do sedentary work.**

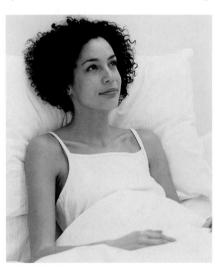

◁ **Don't stay in bed long after you've woken in the morning, but take a few moments to plan the day ahead and visualize it all going really well.**

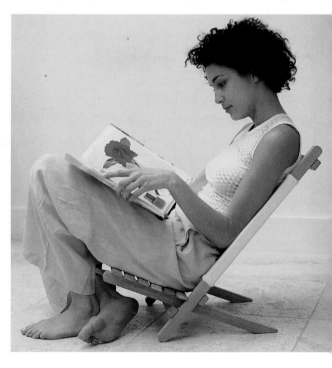

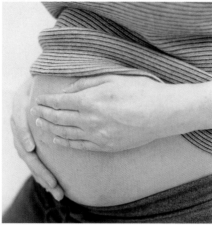

▷ Long before birth a baby is affected by your feelings. Gently massaging your abdomen nurtures the loving bond between you.

pregnancy: glowing with new life

For someone used to being independent, pregnancy is a strange time as a new person's needs start encroaching on a woman's own. Some of the bizarre food cravings a pregnant woman experiences may be her body's attempt to balance her own doshas with the baby's.

The beauty benefits of pregnancy are a welcome side effect: glowing skin, voluptuous breasts and a mane of lustrous hair. Ayurveda can help you keep that glow. In India, a pregnant woman would be massaged by her husband and relatives. Gentle foot and ankle massage, with firm upward strokes, helps relieve swelling. After the fourth or fifth month, oil rubbed into the abdomen helps the skin maintain its elasticity, avoiding stretchmarks, and a backrub can wipe away tension from the face as well as the aching back.

Traditionally, pregnant women were encouraged to snack on sugared hibiscus flowers and rest as much as possible – with one exception: they swept the floors in a squatting position, strengthening the pelvic

area to prepare for childbirth. An antenatal yoga class will teach gentle exercises with the same aim.

Be cautious about massaging the back or abdomen during the early months, in case of miscarriage. Ayurveda recommends plain almond oil: if you want to use anything else, check beforehand with a reputable aromatherapist to find out which oils should be avoided during pregnancy.

If you're taking up yoga, make sure your class is run by a suitably qualified teacher. If you already practise yoga, take advice on how to modify your routine. Remember that not all pregnancies are standard, so seek medical advice if you have any concerns.

▽ You and the baby need to rest. If you haven't got a large Indian family to cosset you, seize time for yourself and accept all the help you can get.

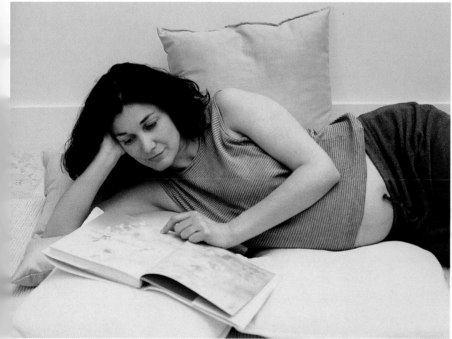

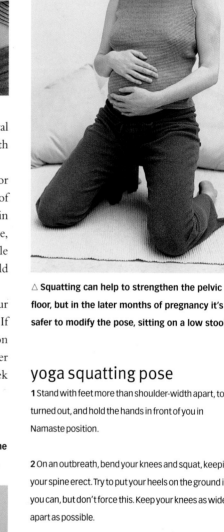
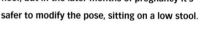

△ Squatting can help to strengthen the pelvic floor, but in the later months of pregnancy it's safer to modify the pose, sitting on a low stool.

yoga squatting pose

1 Stand with feet more than shoulder-width apart, toes turned out, and hold the hands in front of you in Namaste position.

2 On an outbreath, bend your knees and squat, keeping your spine erect. Try to put your heels on the ground if you can, but don't force this. Keep your knees as wide apart as possible.

3 If you've squatted low enough, bring your elbows down between your knees (fingers still pointing upwards), to encourage them further apart. Support your heels on books if they do not reach the floor, and your buttocks on a low stool or rolled towel if you're not comfortable squatting. Eventually you're aiming to put your heels on the floor.

TIPS

• Massage your hair throughout pregnancy and after the birth, to reduce the risk of hair loss caused by hormonal changes.

• Drink hot water with a slice of fresh ginger to relieve morning sickness.

The middle years

As pitta dosha starts to subside and vata increases, women reach the second great transition in life: the menopause. Though pitta is waning, it's no longer regularly reduced by the loss of blood during a period, so it may flare up in sweating and irritability. Heavy periods may be a sign that the body is trying to offload excess pitta. Toxic ama tends to build up as periods become irregular. This leads to lower back pain and an increased risk of growths on the reproductive organs.

Meditation helps combat the stress that magnifies some symptoms and triggers others, such as hot flushes. It's especially important to try to meditate in the morning, to leave the mind calm and able to organize the day's tasks.

Insomnia strikes many women as they reach the menopause. A regular bedtime routine helps to train the mind to turn off at the right time. Ayurveda also recommends going to bed during the kapha hours before 10pm. If this makes you wake up even

earlier, don't spend more than 10 minutes trying to return to sleep – get up and meditate instead.

Yoga practice is also important. Keeping a straight back and open chest allows you to breathe more fully, and weight-bearing exercise keeps bones strong. Add some form of exercise that leaves you slightly out of breath, such as brisk walking or low-impact aerobics. As well as keeping weight under control, this improves the skin.

changing tastes

Choosing the right foods is most important during the menopause, both to bring the doshas into balance and to meet the body's changing needs. Iron, for example, is no longer so necessary, whereas calcium is vital to keep bones strong.

Ayurveda's healthy living rules are made to meet beauty needs as well as promoting long life. The foods that keep the doshas in balance also promote clear skin and a slim, strong physique. Milk and cottage cheese, for example, pacify both vata and pitta while providing calcium and Vitamin D. Base your diet on fresh vegetables and fruit with some dairy foods, nuts, seeds and grains.

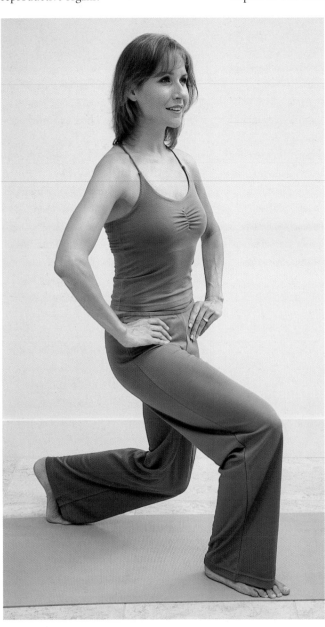

◁ **Staying active keeps you in good shape and slows down the effects of aging. It also eases menopausal symptoms by stabilizing your hormones.**

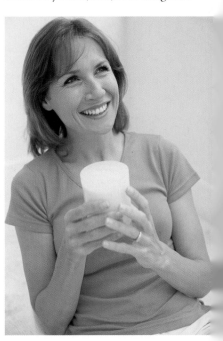

▷ **Changes in your body's hormones can make this stage of your life difficult, but an Ayurvedic remedy will help to balance them.**

ingredients

• 5 almonds

• 3 black peppercorns

• 2 cardamom pods

• 5 ml/1 tsp anise seeds

• 250 ml/8 fl oz/1 cup milk

• 5 ml/1 tsp honey

Soak the almonds in water overnight. Next morning, peel off the skin and grind to a fine paste. Grind the peppercorns, cardamom and anise seeds and mix with the almond paste. Boil the milk, and add your paste and honey. Drink lukewarm.

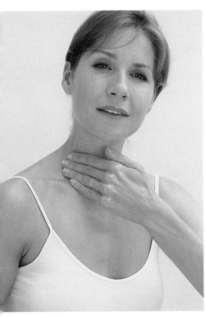

Soothe vata with gentle oil massage, brief steaming and a cooling facepack.

ave your skin

As vata dosha increases with age, its drying influence causes lines, wrinkles and thinning of the skin. Milk, honey and yogurt help to lubricate the skin from the inside, keeping it youthful.

Oiling the skin and then steaming reduces excess vata, making this a suitable beauty treatment throughout life. Because the facial skin can be damaged by too-frequent steaming, it should be done only once or twice a month. Regular use of nourishing facepacks can help to keep the skin properly moisturized, slowing down the aging process.

seeing clearly

Delay the need for reading glasses with some eye exercises. (If you wear contact lenses, remove them first.) Sit with your spine straight and shoulders relaxed, and look straight ahead. Keep your head still while doing the exercises. Hold each eye position for 3–5 seconds and repeat three times.

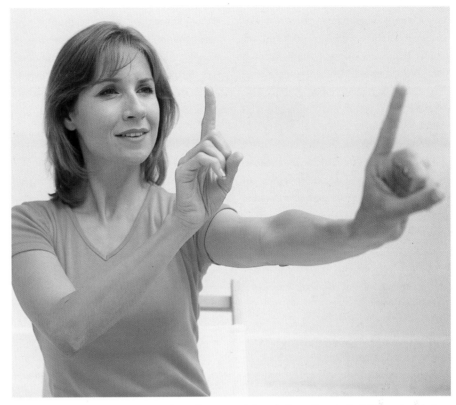

△ **1** With your forefingers at eye-level in front of you, hold one at arm's length and the other half that distance away. Focus on one, then the other.

2 Look diagonally up to the right, then down to the left. Look diagonally up to the left, then down to the right. Look as far as you can up, down, left and right.

3 Rub your hands together to warm them, then cup your palms over your eyes for a few minutes.

NOURISHING MATURE SKIN MASK

ingredients

• 30 ml/2 tbsp oatmeal

• 120 ml/4 fl oz/½ cup milk

• 10 ml/2 tsp olive oil

Mix the oatmeal and milk and simmer until soft. Stir in the oil and mix well. When cool, spread on the face and neck. Leave for 20–30 minutes and rinse with cool water.

TIP

Grate a thumb-sized piece of fresh ginger into a jar of honey and take a teaspoonful a day to slow down the advance of grey hair.

mula bandha: yogic exercise for the pelvic floor

Many women approaching the menopause find their pelvic floor muscles have weakened, giving little or no warning of the need to urinate. Simple exercises can banish this embarrassing problem. Begin by tightening your anus, then add a squeeze in front as if stopping yourself urinating, and hold both squeezes while trying to lift the pelvic floor. It's a tiny movement. If you lay your forefinger flat along the perineum – the strip of skin between vagina and anus – you should feel a very small lift. Start by doing this three or four times after using the lavatory (don't try to stop the flow of urine as this can cause bladder problems), then practise it for 5 seconds at a time, for example while holding any yoga pose.

Moving forward

This is a time when many people – whose earlier lives may have been too hectic for regular practice – discover the benefits of yoga. Notice how much more confidence they have than most older people. This confidence is based on a strength and suppleness that makes them far less prone to accidents and falls.

From as early as the 30s, muscles start to stiffen and joints lose their range of movement. As the years pass, even people with good posture start to walk and turn less smoothly. Long-term yoga practice can delay the onset of these restrictions by many years, but taking up yoga in later life can also reverse some of the changes age has made.

By encouraging correct posture and maintaining flexibility in the spine, it helps to delay the effects of aging. Starting each day with a routine lasting 20–30 minutes leaves you in good shape and gives you time to clear your mind for the day.

▽ Take care of your body, not by reducing activity but by ensuring that all the movements you make are beneficial. Squatting instead of bending, for example, reduces the risk of back pain at any age.

TAKE IT EASY

If you have any medical conditions, check with your doctor before starting any kind of exercise and consider taking a remedial yoga class. In particular:

• Don't do inverted poses such as the Standing Forward Bend and the Downward-facing Dog if you have a blood pressure or heart condition. If you feel at all dizzy in any pose, come out of it gently and sit down.

• If you have arthritis or osteoporosis, beware of poses that put weight on your wrists, such as the Downward-facing Dog.

• Don't do the intense straight-legged bends and backward head-rolls that advanced yoga practitioners carry out. These can injure your spine. In any bend it's better to keep your knees soft, even slightly bent, and concentrate on gently rolling your spine down.

• After a yoga session you should be aware of the muscles you've worked, and may even feel a bit stiff over the next day or so when you're new to the practice. But your joints shouldn't hurt and any stiffness should wear off after a couple of days. If you do experience any pain, stop practising and see your doctor.

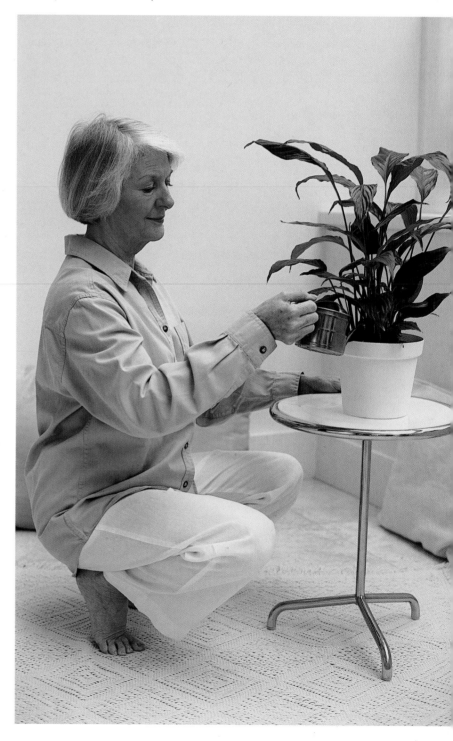

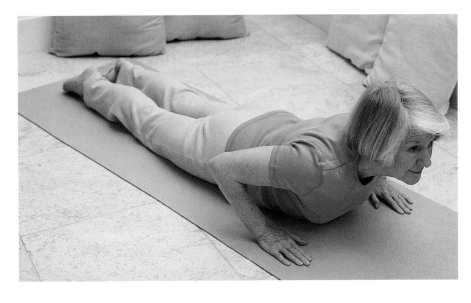

aily yoga routine

ou should include asanas from each of the main roups, to work all parts of the body: standing, tting and lying down; back bends, forward ends and twists. The following is a gentle and ffective series suitable for older beginners.

Warm up by performing the Cat movement several mes to get your spine working.

Stand up in the Mountain pose, to centre you and help eep your balance steady. As people age their sense of alance starts to fade, and it is this as much as loss of rength that leads to potentially dangerous falls. eeping a good sense of balance gives you the same onfident stride you had when you were young.

Move into the Standing Side Stretch. Check that you re breathing naturally and in rhythm with your movements: in as you lean downwards, out as you come p. Return to the Mountain pose and take a moment to eel centred again.

4 Now move into the Standing Forward Bend, eeping your knees slightly bent if you are new to his. If you feel any strain on your back, just move orwards enough to put your hands on a support such as a stable piece of furniture. Concentrate on keeping your back flat and your head in line with your spine.

△ **5** Return to the Mountain pose for a few moments, then lie down on your stomach and move into the Cobra pose. Keep your elbows bent and focus on opening your chest, letting your shoulders sink down and back, away from your ears. When you look upwards, do not to let your head tip back. You're aiming for a natural curve at the neck, without compressing the vertebrae. The same goes for the lower back, don't push yourself up with straight arms and an unnatural arch in your lumbar spine – it's the thoracic vertebrae in your upper spine that need to move.

6 Lower your chest and come smoothly out of the Cobra, then push your hips back and bend forwards into the Child pose, relaxing your spine by letting it curve in the other direction.

7 Move into a kneeling position and into the Dog pose.

8 Next, go into the Bridge, to increase flexibility in your spine. Keep your heels and your arms on the floor, with your palms facing down. You are aiming for a gentle curve in your spine.

9 Roll on to your side and sit up, then move into the Cow pose. This is meant to promote long life, because it opens your chest and stops your lower back stiffening. If you find the leg position difficult, simply sit or kneel with your spine straight.

10 Complete your routine by relaxing for a few minutes in the Corpse pose. Come up by rolling on to your side.

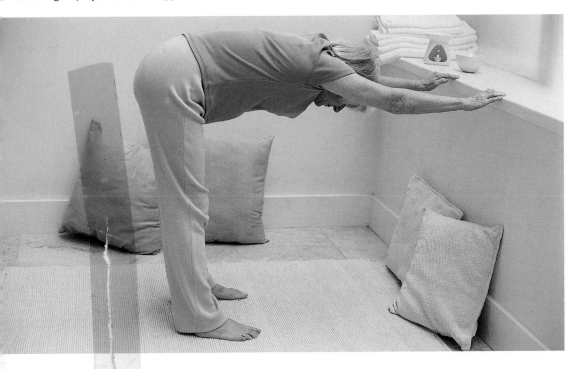

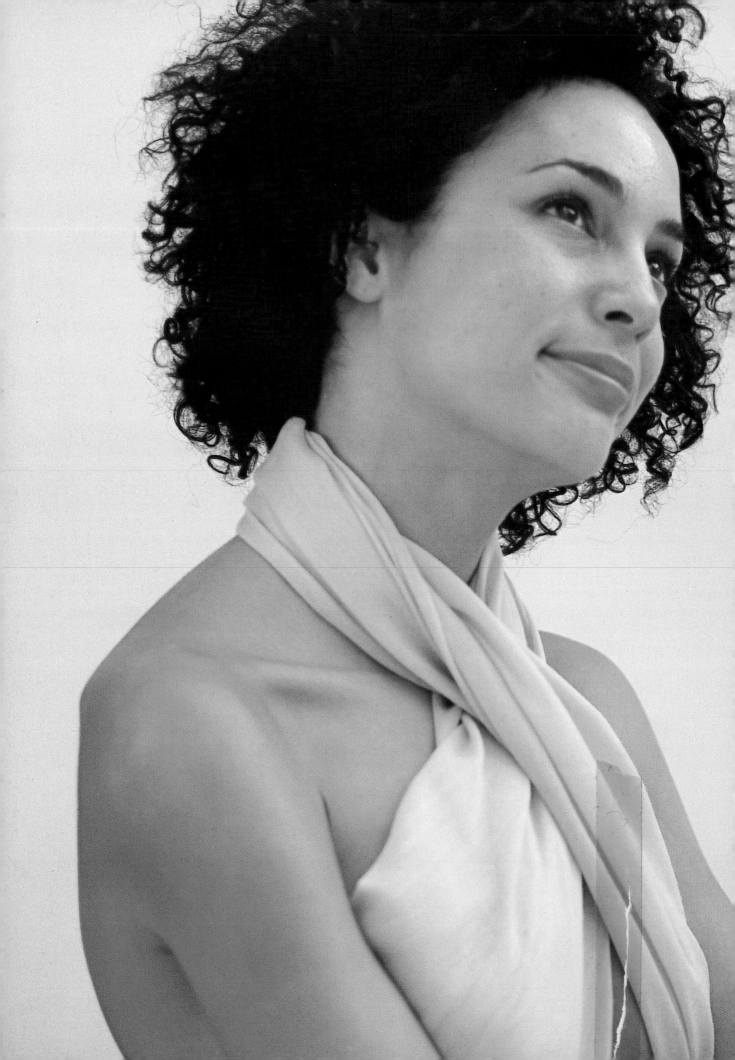

The Food of Life

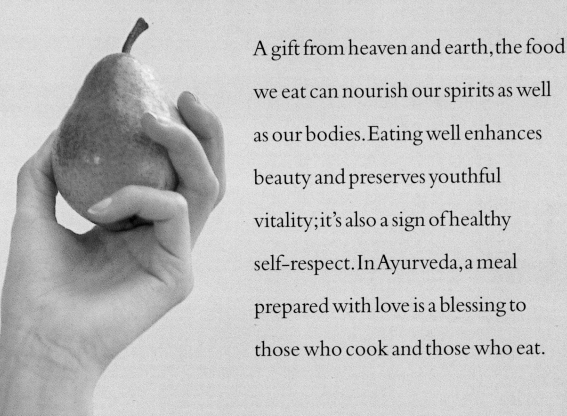

A gift from heaven and earth, the food we eat can nourish our spirits as well as our bodies. Eating well enhances beauty and preserves youthful vitality; it's also a sign of healthy self-respect. In Ayurveda, a meal prepared with love is a blessing to those who cook and those who eat.

Eating well

For many of us, food is at best simply fuel, at worst an enemy. Modern cook books set standards unknown to previous generations, yet most of the food we eat is commercially prepared. Nearly half of us are on a slimming diet at any given time, yet our average weight is rising steadily. No wonder so many of us view food with anxiety.

The Ayurvedic outlook is like a breath of sattvic fresh air. It teaches that eating is a pleasure, and one that does nothing but good. This approach doesn't lead to binge-eating; instead, it means putting a little time and thought into preparing food from fresh ingredients, then savouring it as you eat.

The freshness and quality of the food are important, since unwholesome ingredients create ama, or toxins, in the body. A diet that is based on meat, alcohol, processed foods, dairy products and white sugar and flour produces a lot of ama, leading to disease, bad breath, dull skin and unhealthy hair, while fresh, natural foods give you energy and vitality, and let your natural beauty shine through.

Ayurveda further emphasizes the need to digest food properly, since poor digestion leaves by-products that can also develop into ama. That's why each dosha type needs to eat a slightly different range of foods – those that they're most easily able to digest.

cooking with love

In today's speedy world we often feel too rushed to cook with fresh ingredients. But the steady rhythm of chopping vegetables and stirring pots can create a calm space in the day. And Ayurveda's simple recipes take little time to prepare.

In a traditional Indian household, the kitchen is an almost sacred place. Since everything in creation is deemed to have a soul, everything is entitled to be treated with respect – especially food, which imparts its life force, or prana, to the eater. Followers of Ayurveda believe that the feelings you experience as you cook enter the food and

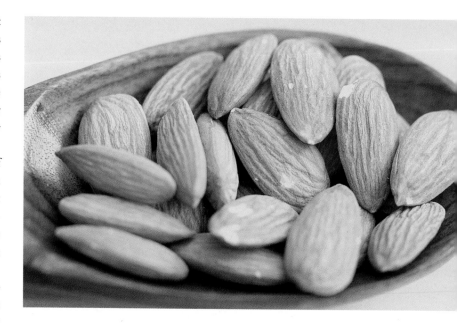

△ To Ayurveda, almonds are full of prana; in Western terms they're rich in Vitamin E, calcium and beneficial fats – either way, a perfect snack

affect anyone who eats it. So don't resent the time you spend cooking. If you enjoy creating a dish, feel nothing but love for those who are going to eat it (including yourself) and look forward to eating it, you'll be endowing the food with health benefits that can't be bought.

food basics

The mainstays of your diet should be fresh fruit and cooked vegetables, grains, nuts and seeds. Add salads and certain animal foods, depending on your dosha. Locally grown organic produce in season is the most natural, as long periods in transport or storage reduce nutritional value.

Meat and dairy produce should be organically produced. Factory-farmed animal foods are risky even by Western standards: they may be diseased or contain drug residues. But such foods are doubly harmful by Ayurvedic standards: the miserable lives of the animals produce low-quality prana, and your action in supporting intensive rearing creates bad karma.

Followers of Ayurveda are frequently vegetarian. Plant foods are full of prana and organic choices are best, as their chemical-free growth causes no harm either to them or to the environment. These are the mo physically and spiritually nourishing food you can find.

how to eat

• Eat at regular times, leaving at least fou hours between meals.

• Don't eat unless you're hungry. If you hav no appetite, wait until your next meal time drinking warm water in between. Bu don't go without food for more than a day.

• Always sit down to eat, and don't watc television, read or have emotiona conversations during the meal.

• Eat slowly and savour food. This stops yo over-eating, since it takes a while for you brain to register that you've eaten enough.

• Try doing a mindfulness meditation whil eating. Focus your attention on the food: it colours, shapes, smell, texture and taste You're less likely to overeat when you mind's on your meal.

• Eat raw fruit alone, not as part of a meal.

• Fast on fruit and vegetable juices and wate for one day a month.

Fresh organic fruit and vegetables are the mainstay of an Ayurvedic diet, good to eat without harming the earth they came from.

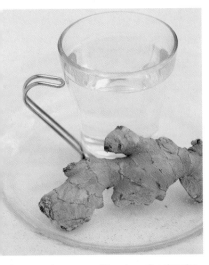

Ginger tea is renowned for strengthening the digestion and alleviating feelings of nausea.

what to drink

Drink enough water to ensure that your urine is always a pale yellow colour: up to 2 litres/3¹/₂ pints a day is beneficial. Warm or hot water is best, and Ayurveda doesn't recommend drinking ice-cold water.

Other healthy drinks are herbal teas, milk (depending on your dosha), fruit juices and vegetable juices.

Ginger tea strengthens *agni*, the digestive fire. Warm water also aids digestion and should be drunk throughout the day.

Choose healthy beverages more often than alcohol or stimulants like tea or coffee.

Cranberry and apple juice are both full of vitamins. Dilute fruit juices with water for the best effects on the body.

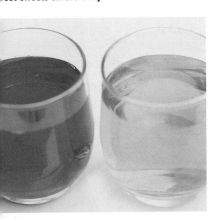

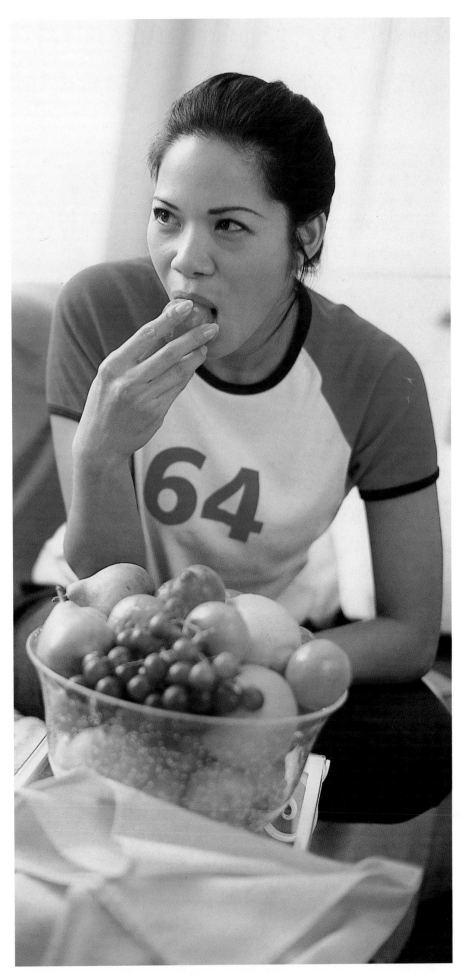

The inner qualities of food

The gunas, or qualities, of foods are as important as their taste and nutritional value. All aspects of nature contain these inner properties – sattva, rajas and tamas – and therefore affect our own gunas whenever we come into contact with them. Since the food we eat becomes part of us, its guna has a particularly strong effect.

sattva

Few people attain the sattvic state of enlightenment, but when we approach it we're fully alert, clear-thinking and compassionate. Sattvic foods, the ones closest to that state themselves, help us towards it. They are the lightest and most wholesome ingredients, close to their

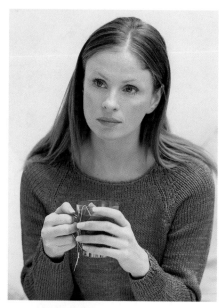

◁ **Light, healthy drinks and foods help you towards the sattvic state, in which you are peaceful and unburdened by negative feelings.**

natural state, such as fresh fruit and vegetables, honey, nuts and whole grain. The lighter dairy products – milk, yogurt and butter – are also sattvic. In keeping with Ayurveda's non-violent ethic, the most sattvic food causes no harm, so the best diet is based on organic fruit and vegetables, locally grown to reduce the environmental costs of transport, and organic dairy produce from animals kept in humane conditions.

rajas

The rajasic state is turbulent, always on the go and easily irritated. Rajasic food is the kind that fuels the go-getting Western world, and each time we eat it it adds to that tendency in us. Rajasic food is not bad because we do need some stimulation, but since Ayurveda values peace more highly than profits, it recommends eating it in smaller quantities. Following that advice will do your body as much good as your soul, since rajasic food is the most likely to cause heartburn. If you have any tendency to be aggressive, cut down on it still further. It's high-protein, high-energy fuel. Rajasic

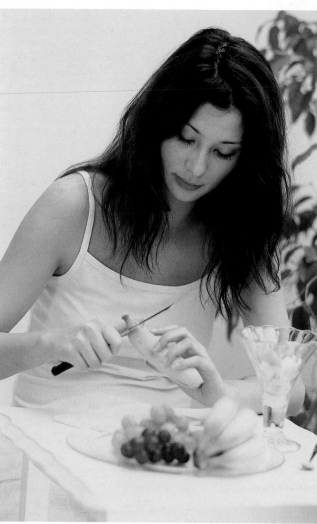

◁ **Fruit pacifies vata and pitta doshas and – especially when cooked – makes a healthy substitute for the cakes and sugary foods that can aggravate kapha.**

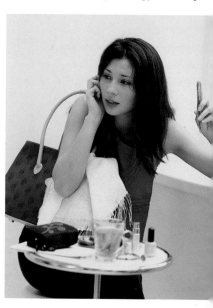

▷ **Rajasic foods fuel the Western lifestyle that leads to stress and burnout. Snacking adds to the ill effects, so take time to eat nourishing food.**

We need high-
protein foods to build
our physical strength
and give us rajasic
energy. They only
cause harm if, as in
the average Western
diet, we eat too much
of them.

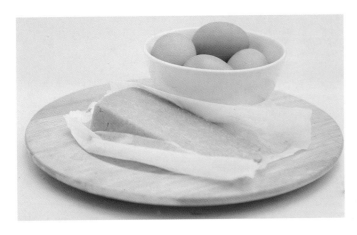

foods include meat, fish, eggs, hard cheese,
hot peppers, sugary foods and root
vegetables, along with anything that has
been fried, pickled or highly spiced.

tamas

The tamasic state of mind is lethargic,
ignorant, selfish and dull. It is fuelled by
processed foods, artificial flavours or
sweeteners, chemical preservatives, factory-
farmed meat and dairy produce, and
anything mass-produced without respect or
made from low-quality ingredients. Meaty
junk food is about as tamasic as food can be.
Food that's stale and has lost its life force is
tamasic too. For this reason, Ayurveda
recommends cooking food fresh every day
rather than using leftovers. Alcohol falls into
the tamasic group, since although it's a
stimulant at first it soon has a dulling effect.

▽ Mass-produced junk food has tamasic effects,
but homemade cakes are a treat: moderation,
quality and individual needs are important.

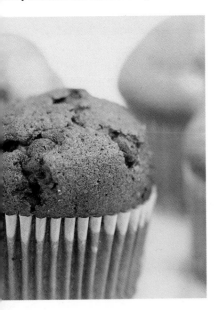

▽ **Alcohol pushes us away from the sattvic state
by causing confusion, damaging health and
promoting aggression and laziness.**

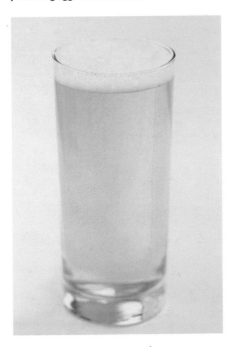

the six tastes

Ayurveda recognizes six flavours, which
affect the balance of doshas. We all need all of
them, but in differing amounts. You don't
need to give up any of your favourite
ingredients completely; if they're in a group
that increases your dominant dosha, just eat
less of them or prepare them in a way that
makes them more suitable, such as tossing
salad in a rich dressing to reduce its vata-
raising properties.

• **Sweet:** increases kapha, reduces vata and
pitta. Sweet-tasting foods such as honey,
cucumber, dried fruit, most fresh fruits, and
foods that become sweet when cooked,
such as apples and onions. High-protein
foods such as meat and nuts. Fats and oils.
Butter, ghee and milk. Rice.

• **Sour:** increases kapha and pitta, reduces
vata. Vinegar, pickles and aged food. Yogurt
and cheese. Tomatoes. Citrus fruits.

• **Salty:** increases kapha and pitta, reduces
vata. Salt, soy sauce.

• **Pungent (spicy):** increases vata and pitta,
reduces kapha. Chillies, sweet peppers,
many herbs and spices.

• **Bitter:** increases vata and reduces pitta
and kapha. Most salad leaves and green leafy
vegetables. Fenugreek and a few other bitter
herbs. Coffee, chocolate.

• **Astringent:** increases vata and reduces
pitta and kapha. Beans, peas, chickpeas,
lentils. Cauliflower, broccoli, fennel,
asparagus, chicory, aubergines (eggplant),
celery, Savoy cabbage. Tea.

GHEE

Clarified butter, or ghee, is not only a
mainstay of Indian cooking but an
important Ayurvedic health product. You
can make your own, though it may not
taste quite the same as the product
bought in Indian shops, which is often
made with yogurt. If you have high
cholesterol and don't normally eat animal
fats, check with your doctor. If you can't
use ghee, substitute vegetable oils.

   To make ghee, put 1 kg/2¼ lb unsalted
organic butter in a heavy pan and heat
slowly, stirring constantly, until melted.
Turn up the heat and let the butter froth for
a few moments, then reduce the heat and
simmer gently, uncovered, for about 30
minutes, until transparent. Skim off the froth
and any impurities and strain through muslin or
cheesecloth, discarding the milky solids. Leave
to cool and store in the refrigerator.

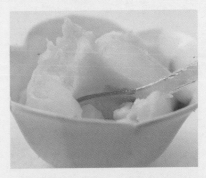

△ **Golden richness with a sweet, nutty taste.**

Diet and your dosha

Each dosha type is pacified or aggravated by different foods, so the food you eat can help to balance your constitution. Try to eat something from each of the six taste groups every day, with most of your intake coming from the groups that pacify your dosha.

the vata diet

Vata is pacified by sweet, sour and salty foods, but aggravated by pungent, bitter and astringent tastes. Raw food tends to increase vata. Try to balance your dry, cool, light constitution with foods that are hot, oily and heavy, such as soups and rich stews. Bananas, grapes and all sweet fruits are good, and meat suits your constitution better than most.

Natural foods are particularly important to vata, since it is aggravated by artificial additives. Most dairy foods suit you, but yogurt is best diluted: try mixing it with water, pure rose water and some honey or chopped fruit, or with water and a little salt to make the Indian drink called lassi.

Though many herbs and spices fall into the pungent category, they're only used in small amounts, so enjoy the warming qualities of spicy foods, though chillies are generally not recommended, since they're considered very dry.

▽ **If it's a hot day but you need to pacify vata, drink a refreshing glass of sweet or salty lassi.**

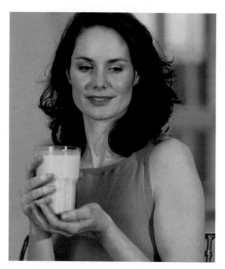

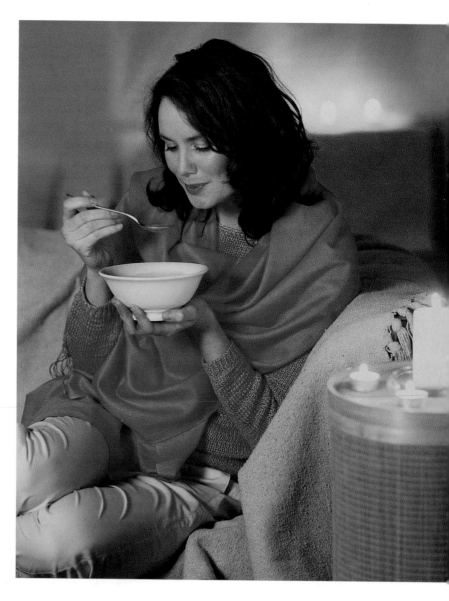

△ **Warmth and comfort soothe excess vata: a cosy room, a quiet evening, a bowl of rich soup.**

Toss salads in mayonnaise or rich dressings containing oil or coconut milk. You can use cooked ingredients to make a warm salad. If you like vegetables from the bitter and astringent taste-groups, cook them with oil or ghee. Ghee will also aid your digestion, which tends to be irregular. Anything light, dry and cool will increase vata, so you should avoid foods like crisps (potato chips), popcorn, dried fruits and undressed green salads.

Though sweet natural foods are good for vata, white sugar and white bread are too dry and light. Alcohol, tobacco and recreational drugs in general have strong vata-inflaming effects and should be avoided altogether or reduced to a minimum.

VATAS COULD TRY…
- Porridge with milk and honey.
- Roasted/stir-fried meat and vegetables.
- Stews cooked with ghee or oil.
- Cooked soft fruit with cream.

the pitta diet

The tastes that help to balance pitta are sweet, bitter and astringent. It is aggravated by those that are pungent, sour or salty. Pitta-pacifying foods are cold, heavy and dry.

Pitta dosha can make you digest your food too quickly, leading to poor absorption. Since Ayurveda teaches that good digestion is the foundation of good health, it is important to strengthen agni, the digestive fire that governs the metabolic processes. Some agni-strengthening foods tend to increase pitta too, but ghee is ideal: it balances pitta while increasing agni. To improve digestion, try to eat slowly in peaceful surroundings at regular times, without overeating. Don't have high-protein food late in the evening. Do take some time to relax after a meal.

Almost all vegetables are good for you, and most fruits that are not sour. Eat plenty of raw food and salad (other than tomatoes). The few vegetables that may not suit you include beetroot, carrots, aubergines (eggplant), garlic, onions and spinach. Chillies, salt and highly spiced food add too much fuel to pitta's fire. Instead, experiment with the cooling tastes of basil, coriander (cilantro), dill, fennel and turmeric, and other mild-tasting herbs. Eat only small amounts of concentrated protein such as red meat, seafood and eggs. Stimulants of all kinds aggravate pitta, so cut down on alcohol and coffee and avoid recreational drugs of any kind.

Excessive pitta heat is cooled by raw foods such as fruit, mild herbs, and vegetables such as broccoli.

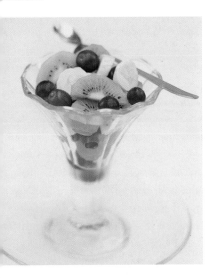

PITTAS COULD TRY...
- Cool stewed apple with pumpkin seeds.
- Green salad with fresh asparagus, drizzled with extra virgin olive oil.
- Rice and beans.
- Ice cream with fresh figs or blackberries.

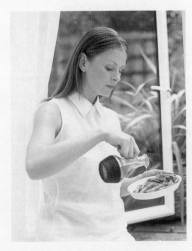

△ **A salad is the ideal pitta lunch.**

the kapha diet

Kapha is balanced by pungent, bitter and astringent tastes, but aggravated by those that are sweet, sour or salty. Foods should be dry, light and hot.

The kapha constitution tends to be cold, so needs warming foods: freshly cooked, spicy or piquant with chillies. Include plenty of vegetables, cooked and eaten hot. Almost all vegetables are good for you, though sweet potatoes can be a little heavy and cucumber has a cooling effect.

You can improve your sometimes sluggish digestion by strengthening agni, the digestive fire. This can be achieved by eating

▽ **Gourmet kaphas can liven up their cooking with chillies, which provide an invigorating heat.**

cloves, pepper (black or cayenne), mustard, cinnamon and horseradish.

The cold nature of salads makes them less suitable for kapha, especially in winter. But don't rule them out completely: choose warm salads, or leaves with a sharp or mustardy taste, but don't smother them in dressing. You have a free hand with almost all herbs and spices, so use these flavourings instead of oils and fats.

Cut down on heavy foods such as wheat, red meat and cheese; lighter alternatives are barley, poultry and cottage cheese. You may have a taste for sweet or salty foods, but these should play only a minor role. Processed foods are high in fat or sugar, and "lite" versions just substitute artificial sweeteners. So leave them on the supermarket shelves and let your natural kapha cooking skills loose on the huge range of real foods.

KAPHAS COULD TRY...
- Cooked buckwheat with cranberries and sunflower seeds.
- Warm salad of raw baby spinach leaves and organic chicken.
- Spicy homemade curries rich with seasonings instead of oil.
- Pears stewed with ginger.

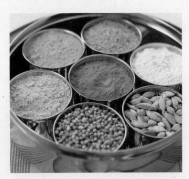

△ **Kaphas can enjoy almost all spices.**

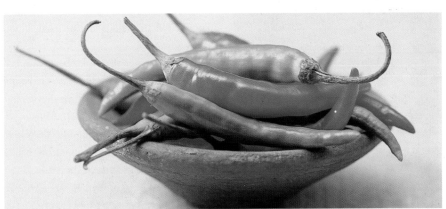

Glossary

The glossary explains all the Ayurvedic terms used in this book. It also includes the names of a number of ingredients used in Ayurvedic treatments; some are Indian herbal remedies, others are familiar foodstuffs that you may encounter under their Indian names if you are buying ingredients from an Indian supplier.

agni fire, transformative force that drives metabolic processes such as digestion.

akhrot walnut.

ama a toxin that can be formed by both physical and non-physical causes, such as indigestible food or painful experiences.

amla/amala/amalaki the Indian gooseberry (*Emblica officinalis*).

arjun/arjuna extract from the bark of the arjun tree (*Terminalia arjuna*).

badam almond.

baingan aubergine, eggplant or brinjal.

besan chickpea or gram flour.

bhasmas medicines traditionally made from precious stones.

bibhitaki extract from the fruit of the beleric myrobalan tree (*Terminalia belerica*).

bindi decorative mark worn on the forehead.

brahmi oil infused with the Indian herb gotu kola (*Centella asiatica*).

chakra one of seven points in the body that draw in energy from the universe.

dalchini cinnamon.

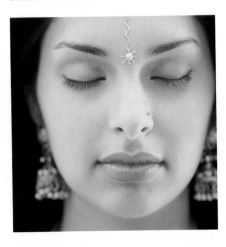

dhania coriander or cilantro.

dinacharya the Ayurvedic daily routine.

diya traditional ghee-burning lamp with a cotton wick.

doshas vata, pitta and kapha, the "flaws" that create each person's individual nature.

ghee clarified butter.

gram flour chickpea flour or besan.

gulab rose petals.

gunas sattva, rajas and tamas, the three inner qualities of all things.

haritaki extract from the fruit of the Indian gall nut (*Terminalia chebula*).

hatha yoga the physical exercises that form a part of yoga.

kapha dosha representing earth and water.

karma the result of our actions in this and previous lives.

kesar saffron.

kokum a sour fruit native to the west coast of southern India, usually available dried.

mahabhutas the five "great elements": earth, water, fire, air and ether (space).

manjishtha/manjista extract from the root of Indian madder (*Rubia cordifolia*).

margosa *see* neem.

marma point place where two kinds of bodily tissue or two different energies meet; prana may become blocked at these points.

mehendi the art of painting the hands and feet with henna.

methi fenugreek.

multani mitti/mati fuller's earth.

Namaste the traditional Indian greeting.

neem Indian tree (*Azadirachta indica*), also known as margosa; all parts are used therapeutically.

ojas the substance that holds body, mind and spiritual levels together.

panchakarma detoxifying procedure that may include enemas and nasal washes.

pitta the dosha representing fire and water.

prakruti the constitution at birth, with all the doshas present in the right balance.

prana the essential life force that circulates in its own invisible system of channels.

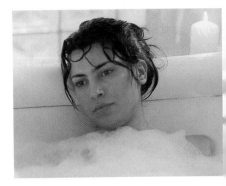

pranayama breathing exercises that form part of yoga practice.

purvakarma preparatory treatments before panchakarma, including steam baths and herbal oil massages.

rajas/the rajasic state the everyday state of mind, in which we may be energetic but are swayed by irritation and emotion.

rasayana treatments aimed at rejuvenation or regeneration.

sattva/the sattvic state the highest and most enlightened state of mind.

shatavari extract from the tuber of wild asparagus (*Asparagus recemosus*).

shikakai Indian soap nut; the ground pods of *Acacia concinna*, used to treat the hair.

shodhana the full detoxifying process, including purvakarma and panchakarma.

sindoor vermilion powder applied to a woman's hair parting during her wedding.

swedana sweat therapy.

tadrak ginger.

tamas/the tamasic state the lowest state of mind: greedy, selfish, violent and dull.

triphala blend of three herbs, amla, haritaki and bibhitaki, to balance the doshas.

tulsi/tulasi holy basil (*Ocimum sanctum*).

ubtan a powder used for skin cleansing.

vata the dosha representing space and air.

vikruti a person's current state, in which health and feelings are affected by the changing balance of the three doshas.

yashti madhu liquorice.

yoga literally "union", a set of spiritual and mind–body practices, including the physical exercises called hatha yoga.

Useful addresses

UNITED KINGDOM
Ayurvedic remedies and treatments
The Ayurvedic Shop
299 King Street
London W6 9NH
Tel: (020) 8563 0303

Neem products
Bioforce (UK) Ltd
Brewster Place
Irvine
Ayrshire KA11 5DD
www.neemco.co.uk

British Wheel of Yoga
25 Jermyn Street
Sleaford
Lincs NG34 7RU
Tel: (01529) 306 851
www.bwy.org.uk

Ayurvedic facelift
Savita Patel
151 Drummond Street
London NW1 2PB
Tel: (020) 7388 9795
e-mail: savita@facelift.fsnet.co.uk

Transcendental Meditation
Freepost
London SW1P 4YY
Tel: (08705) 143 733
www.t-m.org.uk
e-mail: mail@tm-london.org.uk

*Ayurvedic therapies and beauty treatments,
including threading*
Pinka Yusupoff
95 Kenbrook House
Leighton Road
London NW5 2QW
Tel: (020) 7284 4883
e-mail: pinkayusupoff@aol.com

UNITED STATES
American Yoga Association
P. O. Box 1998
Sarasota
FL 34276
Tel: (941) 927 4977
www.americanyogaassociation.org

Ayurvedic treatments, products and training
Ganesha Institute for Ayurveda and
Vedic Studies
4898 El Camino Real, suite 203
Los Altos
CA 94022
Tel: (650) 961 8316
e-mail: info@healingmission.com

INDIA
*Ayurvedic treatments after personal
consultations, products, online courses*
Jiva Ayurvedic Research Institute
1144 Sector 19
Faridabad 121002
Haryana
www.ayurvedic.org

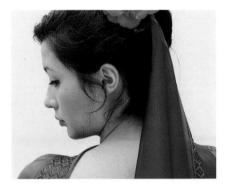

AUSTRALIA
International Yoga Teachers Association
P.O. Box 31
Thornleigh
New South Wales 2120
Tel: (02) 9484 9848
e-mail: info@iyta.org.au

Ayurvedic consultations, products and training
OmVeda Beauty and Health Centre
P. O. Box 248
Rozelle
New South Wales 2039
Tel: (02) 9810 1830
www.omveda.com.au

FRANCE
Ayurvedic products and training
Vedicare
7 Impasse St Pierre
75020 Paris
Tel: 33 (0) 1 44 93 91 26
www.vedicare.net

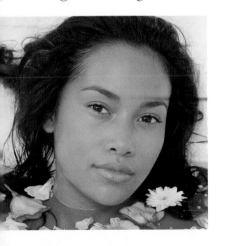

Acknowledgements

Many thanks to all those who contributed information about Ayurveda or traditional Indian beauty care: Moona Baig, Dr Sapna Bhargava, Dr Partap Chauhan, Antony da Costa, Rekha Depala, Claire Laleve, Pratichi Mathur, Savita Patel, Surinder Paul, Seema Rampersad and Pinka Yusupoff. Also to OmVeda for use of their dosha analysis (pp12–13). Special thanks to Yasmin Sadikot, whose vast knowledge of this subject underlies the chapters on skin treatments, for her generosity in sharing it. Special thanks also to Cora Kemball-Cook, for yoga expertise and invaluable friendship, and to David Hall for constant encouragement, love, tea and solidarity.

The publishers would also like to thank: MOT Models agency, the Warehouse studio (setting for location shoots) and Jessica HarrisVoss for being our supple teenage model. Additional pictures: p13br: Simon Bottomley; p47b: Don Last; pp36/7: Alistair Hughes and p66b: Christine Hanscomb.

Index

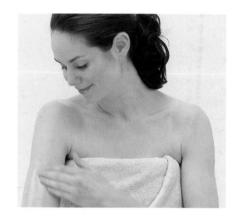

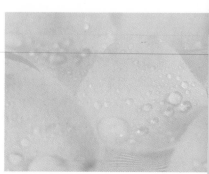